FAST

Stroke Guide

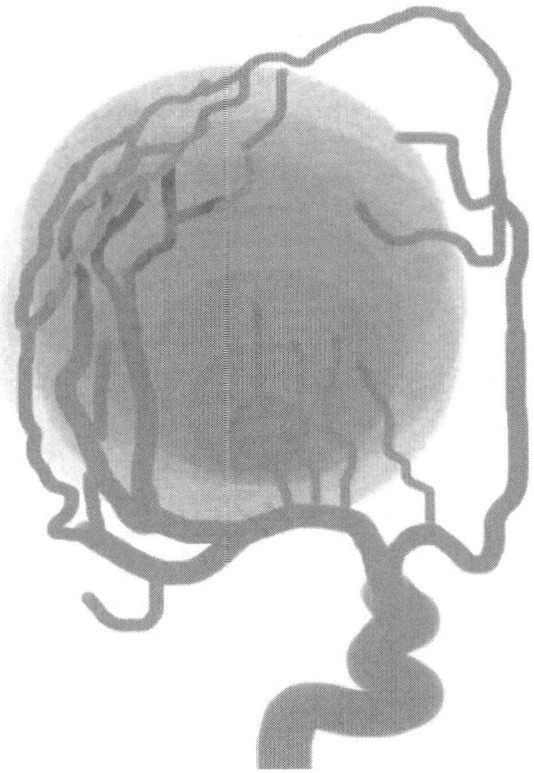

Akram Shhadeh, MD, MBA

ISBN-13: 978-0-578-50083-6

FAST Stroke Guide

First Edition

Akram Shhadeh, MD, MBA
President, Arubah Neuroscience Institute
Interventional Neurology, Stroke, and Neurocritical Care
Cleveland Clinic Indian River Hospital
Vero Beach, FL

Guidance Publishing Company, LLC
Printed in the United States of America

Table of Contents

11. Neuro-angiography Suite and Patient Management During EVT

12. Management of AIS First 24 Hours and After IV tPA and EVT

13. Management of ICH in the First 24 Hours and Anticoagulation Reversal

Preface

"It takes a village!" to save a brain

Stroke is the leading cause of disability and the fifth leading cause of death. Despite the availability of robust treatment for acute stroke, only a small percentage of acute stroke patients receive acute treatment in a timely fashion.

The first FDA approved therapy to reverse stroke symptoms came to life in 1995. The NINDS trial showed significant benefit from administering IV tPA within 3 hours from time of onset. The benefit is greater, and complications are less, the sooner IV tPA is delivered. This new treatment put stroke under light and lots of initiatives were launched to promote early recognition and treatment of stroke. The slogan "time is brain" became very popular amongst healthcare providers.

In 2015, robust positive evidence started emerging about endovascular stroke treatment that expanded the window of acute stroke treatment to include more patients who do not get stroke care due to late emergency room presentation. This treatment specifically targets strokes from "large vessel occlusion"; the most devastating type of ischemic stroke. The new evidence again emphasized the slogan "time is brain".

The slogan "time is brain" is very true and puts huge responsibility on the shoulders of the treating team starting from emergency service personnel, emergency department (ED) physician, neurologist, hospitalist and every single ancillary staff including nurses, technologists, and even transportation.

Acute stroke patients are not only touched by the expert in the field, the stroke doctor. Their journey starts with family and bystanders. This journey is affected by EMS, ED nurses, and doctors' level of understanding of stroke symptoms and urgency. The journey is also affected by many other hospital personnel who perform diagnostic testing required to make treatment decisions. Very often, all the ingredients are available but there is still failure to make the right diagnosis and deliver emergent treatment due to variable level of team members' understanding of stroke.

This book is meant to target all disciplines involved with stroke care and to connect all the dots together to hopefully improve acute stroke recognition, triage, and treatment.
This book is the first published book to attempt to bring all involved parties to a common and consistent understanding of stroke treatment process. The goal is to present all necessary information in a simple, organized, and practical way so that different levels of disciplines (including patient, family, EMS, ED, neurologist, hospitalists, interventionists, and critical care physicians) can understand and implement acute stroke treatment in hopes of reducing acute stroke burden.

I hope you enjoy reading ***FAST Stroke Guide*** and find it a practical resource for patient care.

Akram Shhadeh, MD, MBA

Acknowledgments

I wish to thank my wife, Dr. Asma M. Aouthmany, for her support and tremendous help with editing this book.

I also wish to thank Dr. Amir Batman (emergency room physician) and Dr. Gene Posca (internal medicine physician) for reviewing this book to ensure it is an easy read and useful for all healthcare providers.

1

Brain Composition and Blood Supply

▪ Neurons

The central nervous system (CNS) expresses its sophisticated functions through cells that constitute the nervous system. These cells are very unique in how they work individually and how they communicate with each other. There are two types of cells: *neurons* that are responsible for communication and integration; and *glia cells* that are designed to provide supportive and protective role, but also can modify neurons' function. Our focus in this chapter is on neurons because stroke symptoms are related to neuronal injury.

Neurons consist of three parts that facilitate communication and integration: *dendrites, axons, and axon terminals*. Like any other cell in the body, the neuron has a cell body (soma), which is the center for basic life processes. The neurons communicate with each other and with the rest of the body through electrical and chemical signals (Figure 1.1).

Axons

Each neuron expresses itself through a single axon. Axon is very thin and can be very long. Despite being very long, an

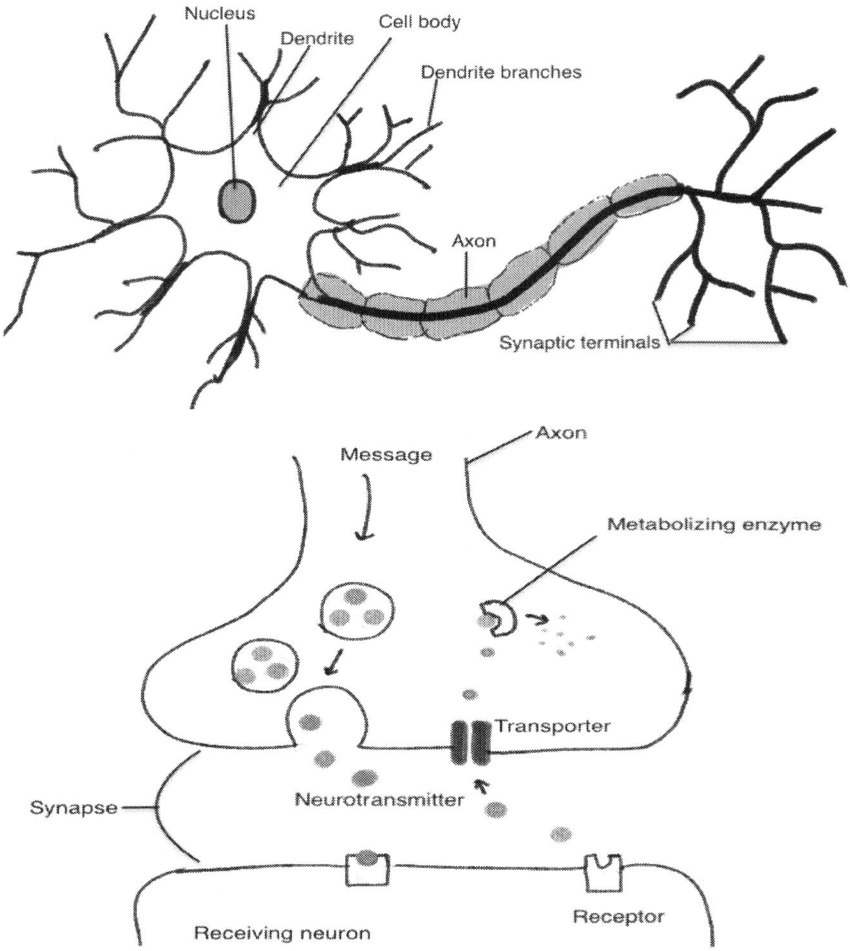

Figure 1.1. A. Neuron consists of a cell body, dendrites and axon. B. Synapse is where neurons communicate with each other by exchanging neurotransmitters.

axon is able to carry information quickly over long distance (communication). An axon ultimately branches to connect with other neurons through axon terminals. Axons carry information (input) from the senses to the CNS (brain and spinal cord), from one part of the CNS to another (coordination), or from the CNS (output) to muscles and glands.

Dendrites

Neurons usually have several dendrites (branches) that deliver input to a neuron. Dendrites are designed both in shape and function to combine information (integration). They act like antennae picking up messages from other nerve cells. They connect to other neurons' body through connections (synapses) and combine the signals they get from these synapses. They have sophisticated bioactive molecules (neurotransmitter molecules) that cross the synapse and fit into special receptors on the receiving neuron body. This leads to stimulation of the receiving cell in different ways to pass on the message [1].

Neuronal ischemic injury

Neurons survive minute to minute on a constant supply of oxygen and glucose carried by blood flow. Blood flow disruptions with resultant instantaneous drop in oxygen and glucose supply causes energy depletion (due to ATP reduction) and resultant loss of function. Drop in supply also has deleterious effect on basic structure and viability of the neurons through excitotoxic mechanisms that include activation of glutamate receptors and release of excess glutamate in the extracellular space. This induces neuron depolarization and dramatic increase of intracellular calcium which in turn activates multiple intracellular fast death pathways (necrosis, fast death). Excitotoxicity also causes apoptotic cell death (apoptosis, slow death). Both necrotic and apoptotic neurons cease to function; however, only apoptotic neurons can resume function when blood flow is re-established. Neurons can regenerate axons but cannot regenerate cell body that is already necrotic [2].

Glia cells

Glia cells constitute about 80% of brain cells and are responsible for most types of brain tumors. Their main function is to provide nourishment, protection, and structural support. Due to the abundance of glial cells compared to neurons, brain imaging modalities can mainly detect changes in brain when pathology affects glial cells in addition to neurons. However, when injury affects only neurons, brain imaging will likely be unremarkable. Thus, negative brain imaging does not rule out neuronal injury. There are different types of glial cells with different functions.

Astrocytes control the blood-brain barrier (gate keeper), transporting useful nutrients and molecules to neurons and blocking harmful ones. They contribute to homeostasis, defense and repair, scar formation, and can affect electrical impulses.

Oligodendroglia are responsible for insulating axons by using a product composed of fatty substance (myelin). Myelin also helps electrical messages to travel faster.

Ependymal cells line the cavities within the brain (ventricles) and secrete protective fluid (cerebrospinal fluid, CSF).

Microglia are the main immune cells in CNS. They protect the brain from invaders and cleanse debris. They can also prune synapses.

Brain anatomy and function

The CNS is composed of the brain and spinal cord. The peripheral nervous system (PNS) consists of nerves that originate in the spinal cord and cranial nerves that originate mainly from brainstem. The brain resides within the skull and is divided into the cerebrum, cerebellum, and brainstem (Figure 1.2). The brain does not have the ability to regenerate lost areas, so any loss of brain tissue usually has permanent impact on patients and families.

Cerebrum

Cerebrum is composed of right and left hemispheres. It is located in the front compartment of the skull (anterior and middle fossa). It is the largest part of the brain because it is the center for higher functions such as speech, reading, learning, initiation of coordinated movement, hearing, vision and many other cognitive functions.

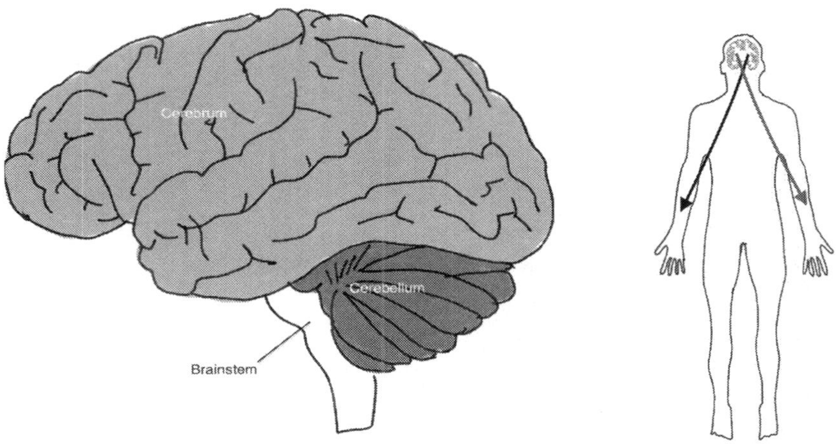

Figure 1.2. The brain consists of cerebrum, cerebellum, and brain stem. Each hemisphere controls the opposite side of body. The axons (motor and sensory; the motor fibers are demonstrated) cross in brainstem.

The cerebral hemispheres have grooves (fissures), which divide the brain into multiple areas (lobes). There are 4 lobes: frontal, temporal, parietal, and occipital. Each lobe may be further divided by shallower groves (sulci), and into different functional areas (gyrus). These lobes have complex inter-relationships across each other and across both hemispheres (Figure 1.3).

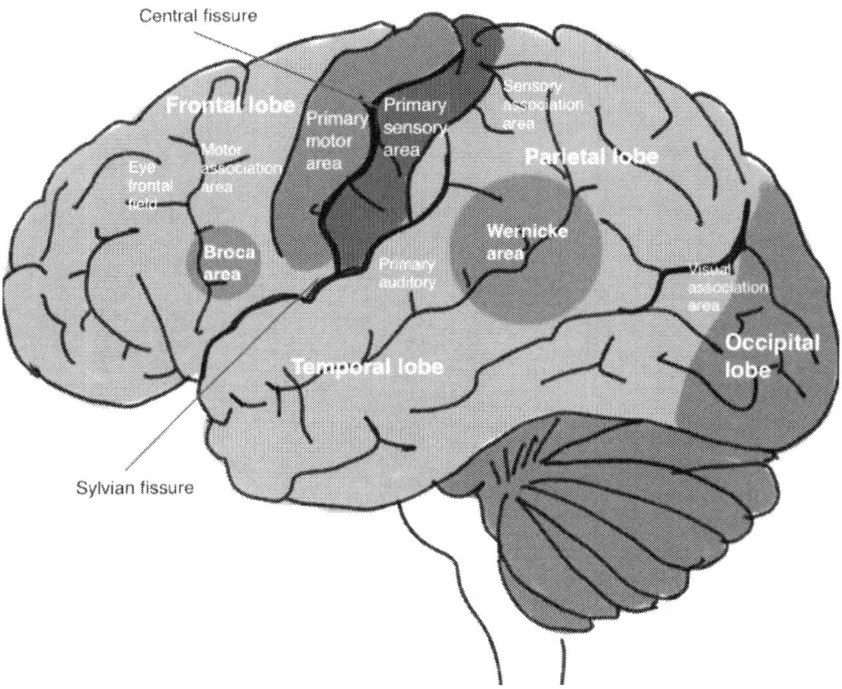

Figure 1.3. The lobes and functional areas of the cerebrum.

Communication signals travel from one gyrus to another, from one lobe to another, from one side of the brain to the other, and to deeper structures. The function of each lobe is explained further in chapter 3. Table 1.1 shows the very basic function of each lobe.

Deep structures of the cerebrum

Hypothalamus is the main control station of the autonomic system (such as temperature and blood pressure) and basic behavioral functions such as thirst, hunger, sexual response, emotions and sleep cycle. It also has a major role in regulating hormones.

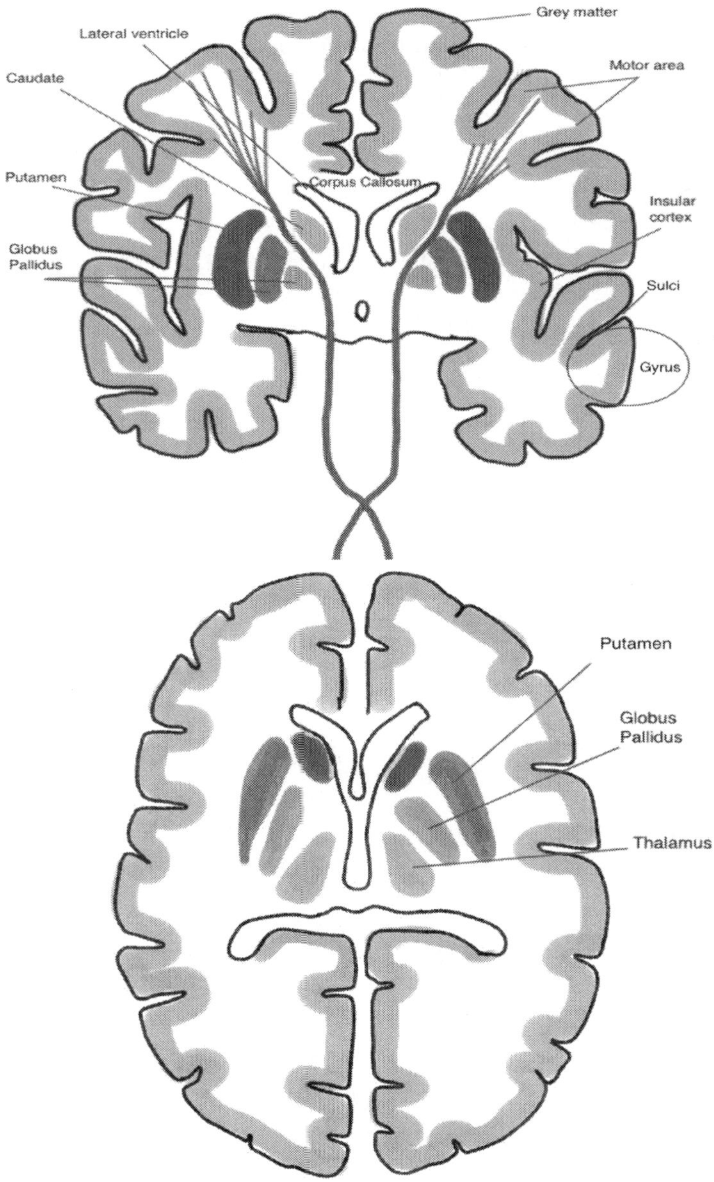

Figure 1.4. Coronal and axial cross-section showing the basal ganglia.

Thalamus is the relay station for almost all input and output signals into and from the cortex. It has also primary role in pain sensation, alertness, memory, and attention.

Basal ganglia work with the cerebellum to coordinate fine motions, such as fingertip movements. It includes the caudate, putamen and globus pallidus (Figure 1.4).

Limbic system is the center of memory, emotions and learning. It consists of cingulate gyri, hypothalamus, amygdala (emotional reactions) and hippocampus (memory) (Figure 1.5).

Pituitary gland is the master of glands. It lies in a small pocket in the skull base (sella turcica). It is connected to the hypothalamus and together they control most endocrine glands.

Pineal gland is located behind the third ventricle. It secretes melatonin to regulate the body's biologic clock and circadian rhythms.

Brainstem

Brainstem connects the cerebellum and cerebrum to the spinal cord. It is the most important part of the brain because it hosts the "life center" which regulates basic life functions. It also houses the ascending and descending cables (tracts) between the spinal cord and brain; basic reflex centers (respiratory, cardiovascular system); and consciousness center. It consists of three parts (midbrain, pons, medulla). It also contains the neurons (nuclei, generator) of most of the cranial nerves (Table 1.2).

Midbrain connects the pons and medulla to the cerebrum. It mainly contains the nuclei of the arousal nerves (reticular formation), oculomotor nerves (3; controls most eye movement), and trochlear nerves (4; controls downward and inward eye movements) in addition to Edinger Westphal center (controls pupillary reaction) (Figure 1.6a).

Pons connects the midbrain to the medulla. It mainly contains the nuclei of the trigeminal nerve (5; controls face sensation and chewing muscle), abducens nerve (6; controls outward eye movement), facial nerve (7; controls facial muscles), and cochlear / vestibular nerve (8; controls hearing and balance) (Figure 1.6b).

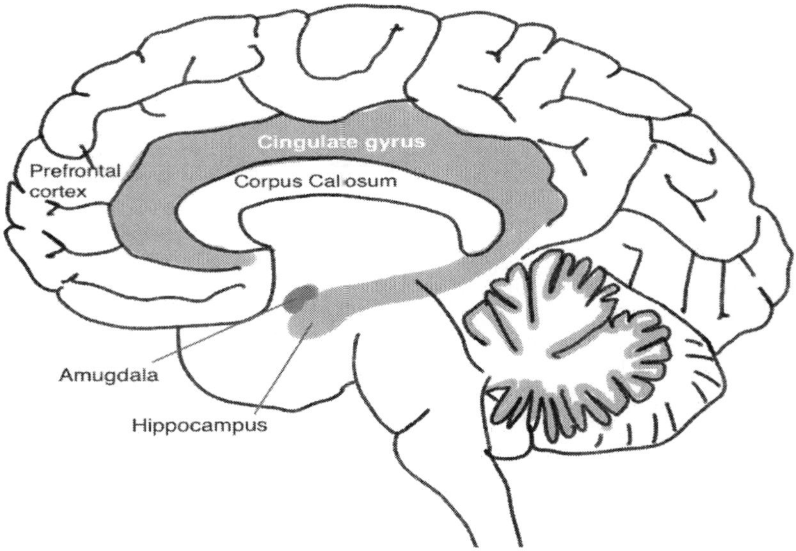

Figure 1.5. The limbic system mediates memory formation. Recent events (short-term memory) is coded in prefrontal cortex. Older events (long-term memory) is coded in the hippocampus.

Medulla connects the pons superiorly to the spinal cord. It mainly contains the nuclei of the glossopharyngeal nerve (9; controls swallowing, throat sensation and taste), hypoglossal nerve (12; controls tongue), vagus nerve (10; controls autonomic function) and accessory nerve (11; controls some of neck and shoulder muscles nerves) [3] (Figure 1.6b).

Most of these cranial nerves, except for 2, control the respective function on the same side of the body. This feature helps distinguish brainstem stroke clinically from other cortical and subcortical strokes.

Table 1.1. Basic functions of cerebral lobes.

Function of brain lobes	
Frontal lobe	Reasoning, planning, parts of speech (expression), movement, emotions, and problem solving
Parietal lobe	Orientation, recognition, perception of sensory stimuli
Temporal lobe	Perception and recognition of auditory stimuli, memory, and speech (reception)
Occipital lobe	Visual processing

Table 1.2. Basic function of cranial nerves.

Function of Cranial Nerves		
I	Olfactory	smell
II	Optic	sight
III	Oculomotor	moves eye, pupil
IV	Trochlear	moves eye
V	Trigeminal	face sensation
VI	Abducens	moves eye
VII	Facial	moves face, salivate
VIII	Vestibulo-cochlear	hearing, balance
IX	Glosso-pharyngeal	taste, swallow
X	Vagus	heart rate, digestion
XI	Accessory	moves head
XII	Hypoglossal	moves tongue

Cerebellum (4)

Cerebellum is located under the cerebrum (posterior fossa). The vertical organization is similar to the cerebrum.

Cerebellar cortex is also made of gray matter that is folded into sulci and folia. White matter fills the deeper portion and contains

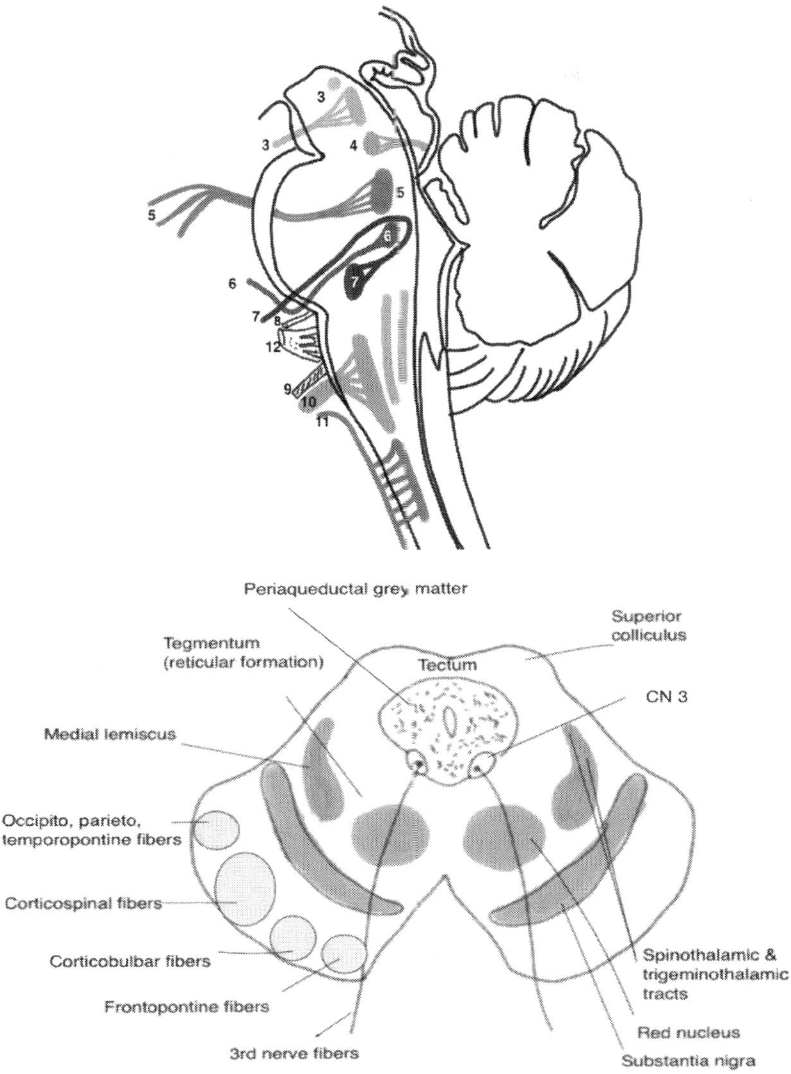

Figure 1.6 a. Brainstem and cranial nerves (top picture) and midbrain (lower picture).

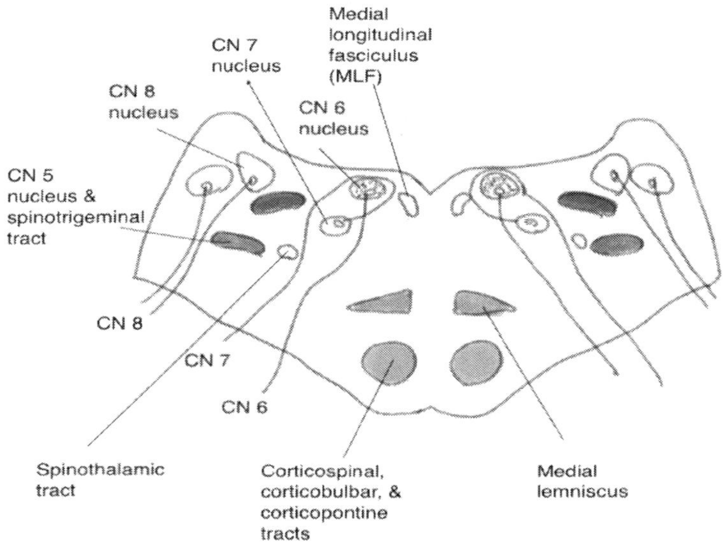

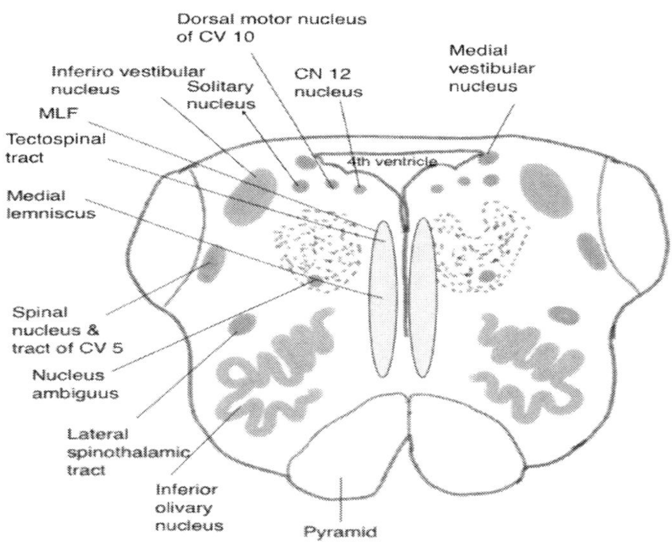

Figure 1.6 b. Pons (top picture) and medulla (lower picture).

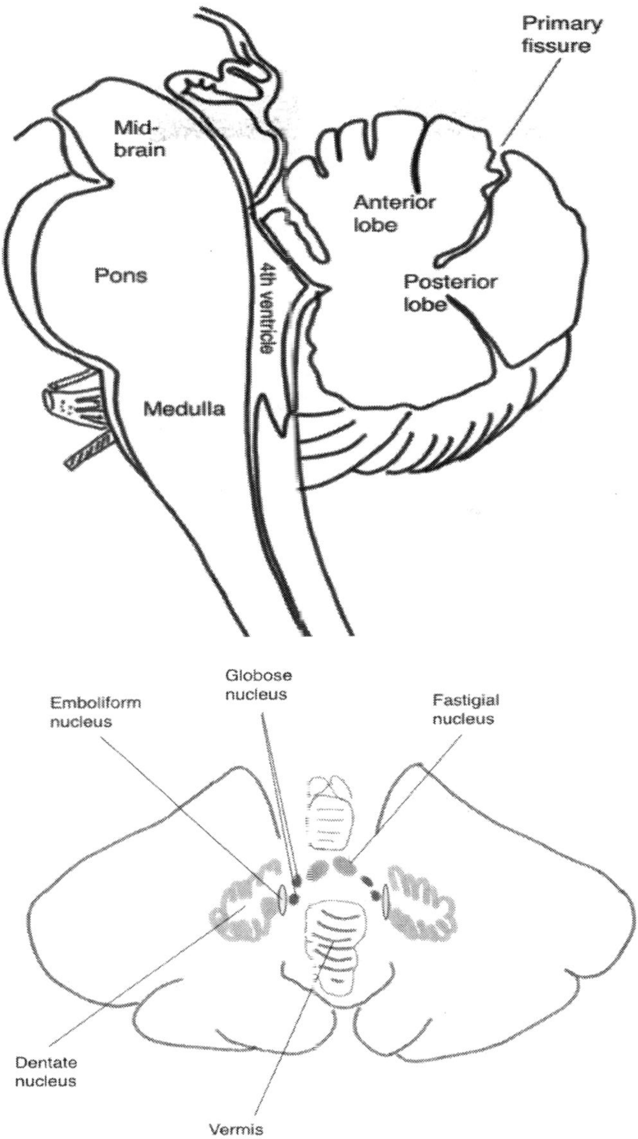

Figure 1.7. Cerebellar sections (top picture) and cerebellar nuclei (lower picture).

the cerebellar nuclei (vestibular, fastigial, interpositus, dentate) (Figure 1.7). From a functional standpoint, there are three distinct regions:

Vestibulocerebellum (flocculonodular) receives afferents (inputs) from the vestibular nuclei and visual cortex through nuclei of the pons and their efferents (outputs) go straight to the vestibular nuclei. It is responsible for controlling and regulating balance and eye movements [(4)].

Spinocerebellum (cerebellar cortex):

> *Vermal* portion receives somatosensory afferents from the spinal cord, vestibular, visual and acoustic and sends its efferents through the fastigial nucleus. It coordinates muscle movement of the head, trunk, neck and proximal portions of limbs [(4)].
>
> *Paravermal* portion receives somatosensory afferents from the spinal cord and trigeminal sensory nucleus and sends efferents through the interpositum nucleus. It coordinates movement of the distal portions of the limbs [(4)].

Cerebrocerebellum (lateral cerebellar hemispheres) receives afferents from most of the neocortex (cerebrum) through the pons nuclei. It sends efferents that reach the thalamus through the dentate nucleus, and then to the cerebral cortex. It performs cognitive functions (visuospatial perception, language processing and modulation of emotions), general planning of motor activities, and motor sequence learning [(4)].

▪ Ventricles and cerebrospinal fluid (CSF) (Fig. 1.8)

The brain has fluid-filled deep spaces (the ventricles) which contains the choroid plexus, a structure that produces protective fluid. This fluid (cerebral spinal fluid; CSF) flows within and around the brain and spinal cord to help cushion it from injury. CSF is constantly being produced by choroid plexus and absorbed from subarachnoid space to the sagittal sinus through arachnoid villi.

A strict balance is preserved between the production and absorption of the CSF to maintain good cushion without increasing ICP. Any disruption or obstruction in the system would shift balance and promote build-up of CSF resulting in enlargement of the ventricles (hydrocephalus).

▪ Skull

The skull is formed from 8 bones that fuse together along suture lines. These bones include the frontal, parietal (2), temporal (2), sphenoid, occipital and ethmoid. The face is formed from 14 paired bones including the maxilla, zygoma, nasal, palatine, lacrimal, inferior nasal conchae, mandible, and vomer.

Inside the skull are three distinct areas: anterior fossa, middle fossa, and posterior fossa (Figure 1.9).

The arteries, veins, and nerves exit the base of the skull through holes called foramina. The foramen magnum is where the spinal cord exits.

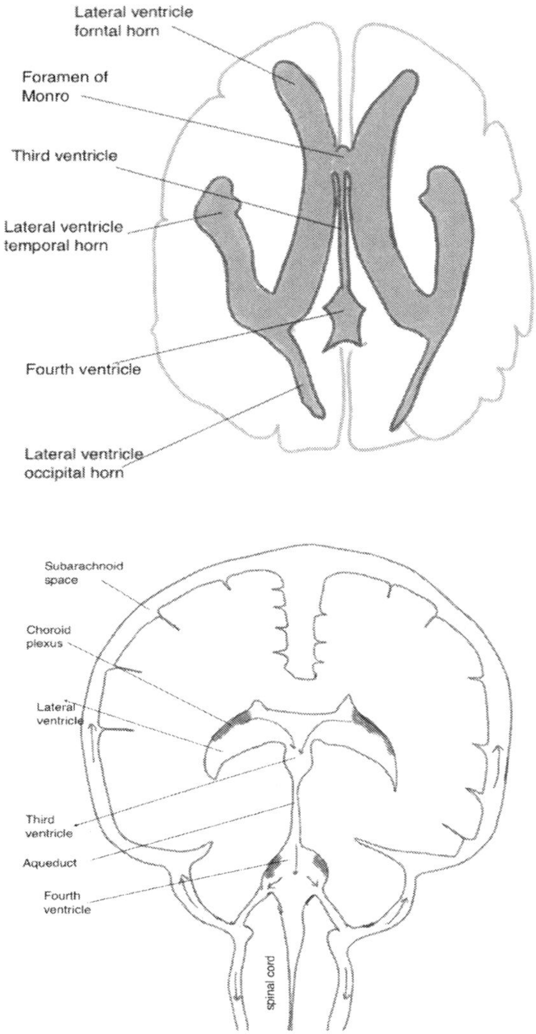

Figure 1.8. CSF is produced in lateral ventricles (from choroid plexus). CSF circulates inside the brain and spinal cord and then outside to the subarachnoid space. Obstruction at any level (foramen of Monro and aqueduct of Sylvius leading to "obstructive hydrocephalus" or subarachnoid space leading to "non-obstructive hydrocephalus") can lead to increased intracranial pressure.

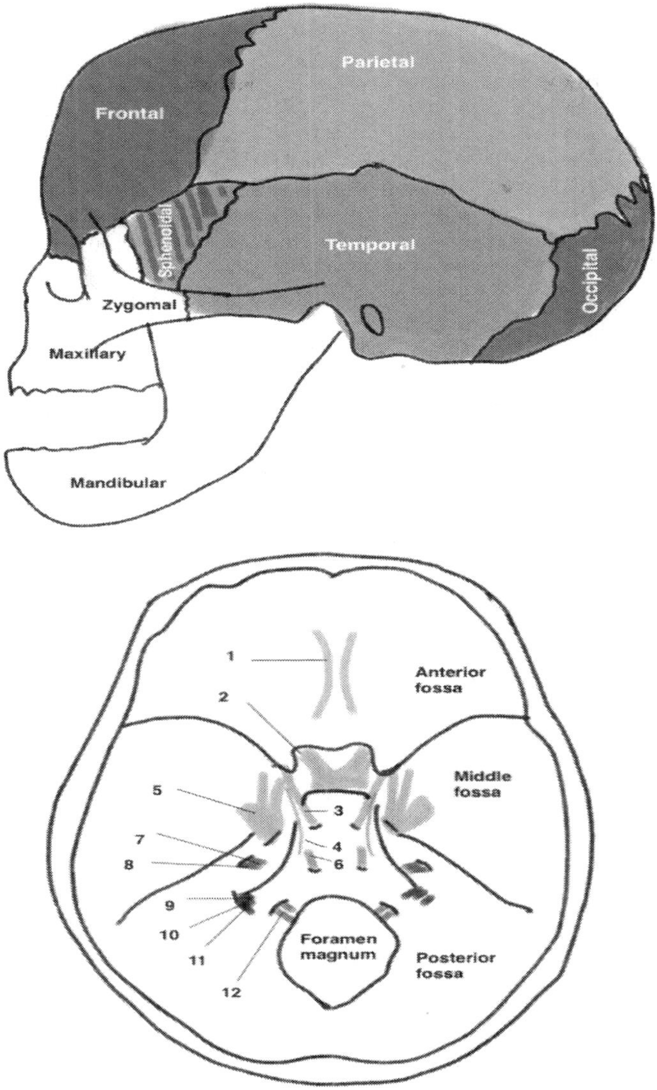

Figure 1.9. The brain is protected inside the skull. The skull is formed from eight bones. The base of the skull is divided into 3 regions: anterior, middle and posterior fossae. All cranial nerves exit from skull base through multiple foramen. After originating from brainstem, cranial nerves exit the skull through multiple foramina. The brainstem exits the skull through the foramen magnum.

Meninges

The brain and spinal cord are covered and protected by three layers of tissue called meninges. From the outermost layer to inward they are: the dura mater, arachnoid mater, and pia mater.

Dura mater is a strong membrane that lines the skull. Its two layers, the periosteal and meningeal dura, are fused and separate only to form venous sinuses. The dura creates little folds or compartments. There are two special dural folds, the falx and the tentorium. The falx separates the right and left hemispheres of the brain and the tentorium separates the cerebrum from the cerebellum.

Arachnoid mater is a thin membrane that covers the entire brain. The space between the dura and arachnoid membranes is called the subdural space.

Pia mater hugs the surface of the brain following its folds and grooves. The pia mater has many blood vessels that reach deep into the brain. The space between the arachnoid and pia is called the subarachnoid space. It is here where the cerebrospinal fluid bathes and cushions the brain.

Blood supply and vascular physiology

To ensure uninterrupted cerebral circulation to the vulnerable neurons, the brain attracts 15-20 % of the cardiac output and it has robust network of cerebral arteries supplying the brain to keep cerebral blood flow of 750 ml/minute. The cerebral circulation is so sacred that there are many safety mechanisms to ensure constant blood supply including autoregulation of the blood vessels.

Brain circulation is divided into anterior (that supply most of the cerebrum) and posterior (that supply brain stem, cerebellum and back part of the cerebrum, the occipital lobe). Anterior circulation is supplied by carotid arteries and posterior circulation by vertebral arteries (Figures 1.10, 1.11 and 1.12).

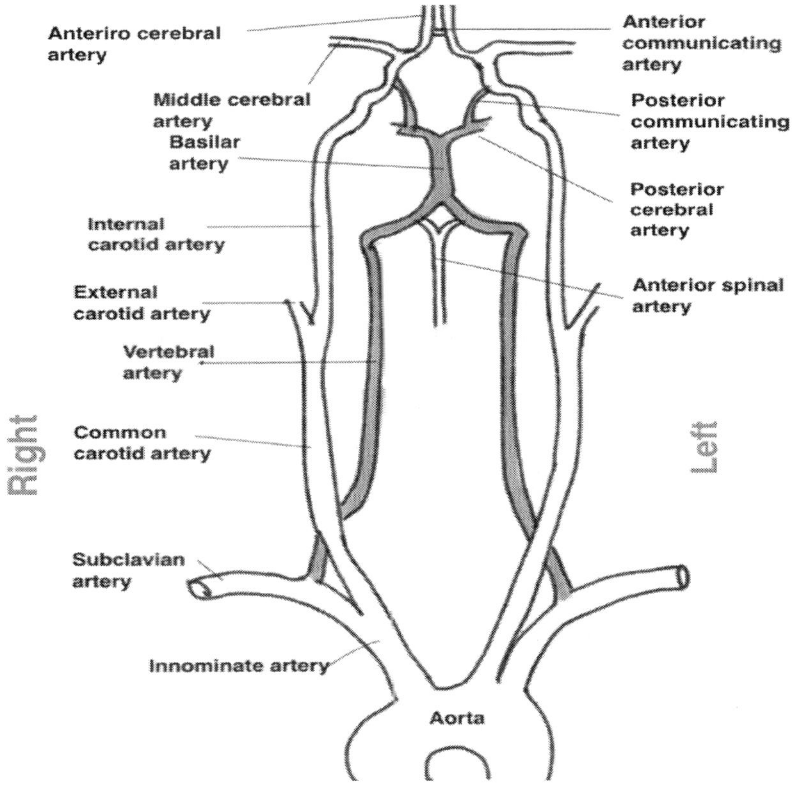

Figure 1.10. The aorta gives origin to the innominate artery which gives origin to the right common carotid artery. The left common carotid artery originates directly from aorta in most individuals. Both common carotid arteries course up the neck and divides into the internal and external carotid arteries. The brain's anterior circulation is fed by the internal carotid arteries and the posterior circulation is fed by the vertebral arteries. The two systems connect at the Circle of Willis.

Anterior and posterior circulations usually connect through the posterior communicating artery on both sides. These two arteries are part of the circle of Willis, which also provides interconnections between both sides of anterior circulation through anterior communication artery.

Anterior cerebral circulation

Internal carotid artery (ICA) branches from the common carotid artery (CCA) in the neck near the jaw corner. It travels vertically through the neck without providing any branches until it enters the skull, as opposed to the external carotid artery (ECA) which provides branches to supply the face, tongue, nose, and throat. The internal carotid artery branches by order into the ophthalmic artery (OA), posterior communication artery (PCOMA), anterior choroidal artery (ACHA), anterior cerebral artery (ACA) and continues as the middle cerebral artery (MCA) (Figure 1.11).

Anterior cerebral artery (ACA) mainly supplies the inner (medial) aspects of the frontal and parietal lobes and basal ganglia.

Anterior communicating artery (ACOMA) is very short artery that connects both anterior cerebral arteries and is part of the circle of Willis. In rare occasions, the ACOMA is absent.

Middle cerebral artery (MCA) forms after branching of the ICA. It travels outward (laterally) and then upward along the convexity of the brain. The MCA can be divided into 4 parts:

- M1 is the first horizontal segment that extends straight and gives many small perforators that supply the basal ganglia.
- M2: there are usually 2 branches that originate from the terminal portion of M1; one extends to the front (anteriorly,

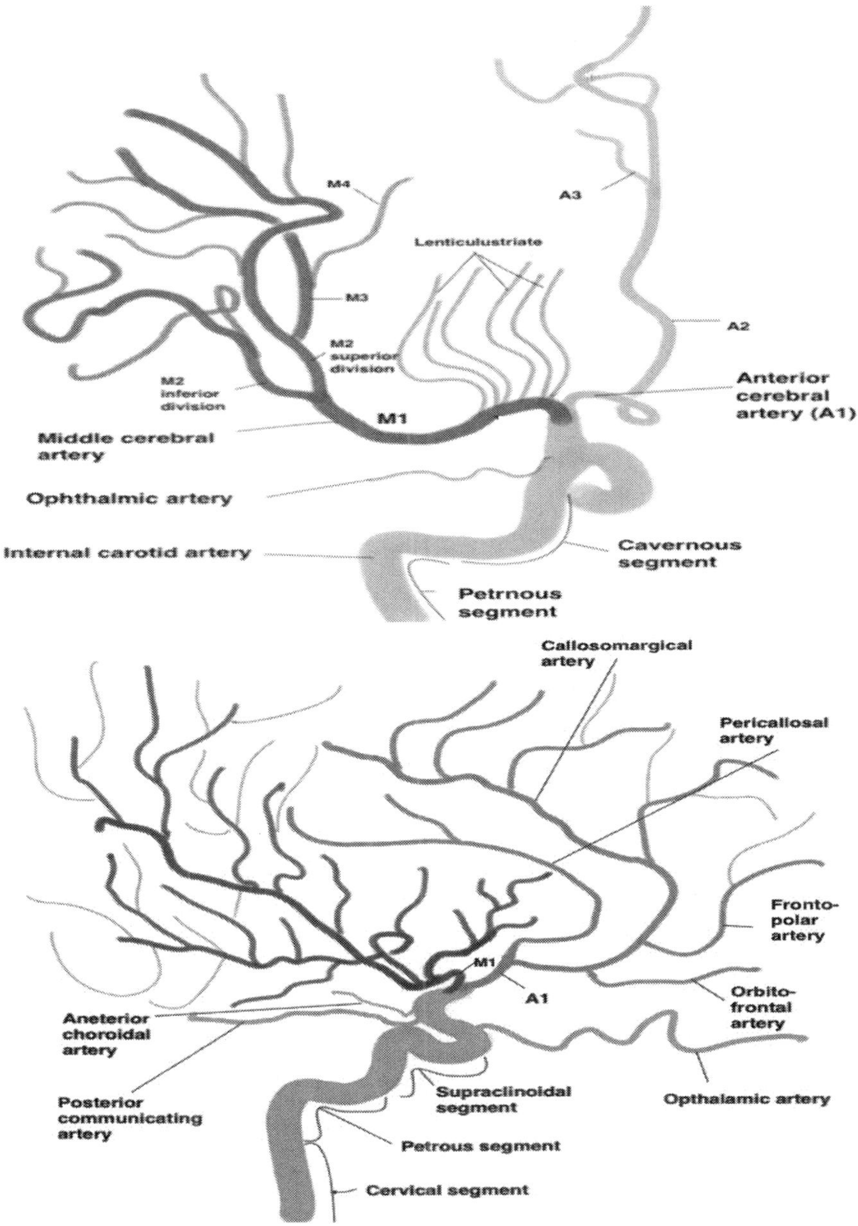

Figure 1.11. Anterior circulation branches (AP view, upper and lateral view).

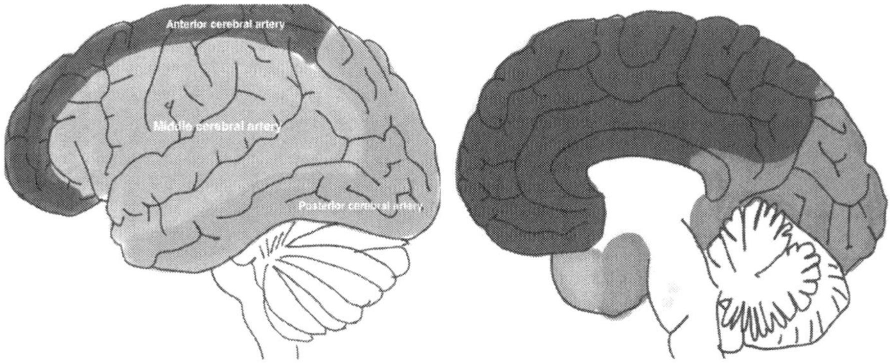

Figure 1.12. Brain anterior vascular territories (lateral and medial aspects).

anterior division); the other M2 branch extends to the back (posteriorly; posterior division).

- M3s are the smaller branches that originate from each of the M2 segments.
- M4s are final terminal or cortical branches that actually reach to the cortical area and gives smaller branches the supply the cortex directly.

Posterior cerebral circulation

The posterior cerebral circulation is the blood supply to the posterior portion of the brain, including the occipital lobes, cerebellum, and brainstem (Figure 1.13). It is supplied by the following arteries:

Vertebral arteries (VA) are branches from the subclavian arteries which primarily supply the shoulders, lateral chest and arms.

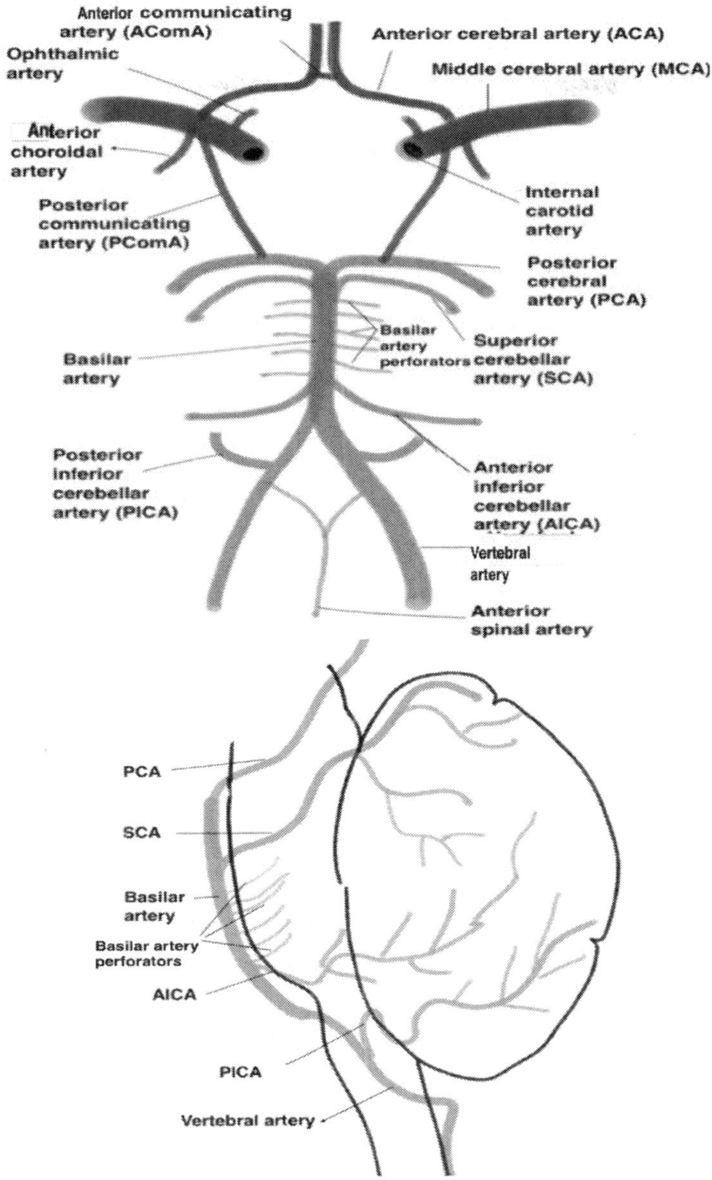

Figure 1.13. Posterior circulation branches and how they form Circle of Willis with anterior circulation (top picture) and how it supplies brain stem and cerebellum (lower picture).

After traveling through the spine, both VAs enter the skull and shortly afterward fuse into the basilar artery (BA). Shortly before forming BA, each VA gives origin to the *posterior inferior cerebellar artery (PICA)* which supplies the outside (lateral aspect) of the medulla in addition to inferior lateral portion of cerebellum.

Basilar artery (BA) supplies the midbrain, cerebellum, and usually ends with two posterior cerebral arteries. During its course, it gives origin to the following arteries:

Anterior inferior cerebellar artery (AICA) is the first direct branch of the basilar artery and it supplies the lower (inferior) portion of the cerebellum.

Pontine branches are very small direct branches of the basilar artery and they supply the superficial and deep portions of the pontine.

Superior cerebellar artery (SCA) is a branch of the basilar artery which supplies the upper (superior) portion of the cerebellum.

Posterior cerebral artery (PCA) supplies the lower inferior part of the temporal lobe, and many other deep structures such as the thalamus and the back portion (posterior) limb of the internal capsule.

Posterior communicating artery is a short artery that connects both posterior cerebral artery and internal carotid artery and is part of Circle of Willis.

▪ Venous drainage

There are two venous drainage systems for the brain: superficial and deep (Figure 1.14).

Superficial venous drainage

The superficial system consists of large dural venous sinuses that are located on the surface of the brain. The largest sinus is the *superior sagittal sinus* that is located under the midline of the cerebral vault. It travels backward and downward to the *confluence of sinuses,* where the superficial system meets deep system. Then the blood drains outside the skull through two *transverse sinuses* that travel outward and downward and form an S-shaped *sigmoid sinus* that connects directly into jugular veins.

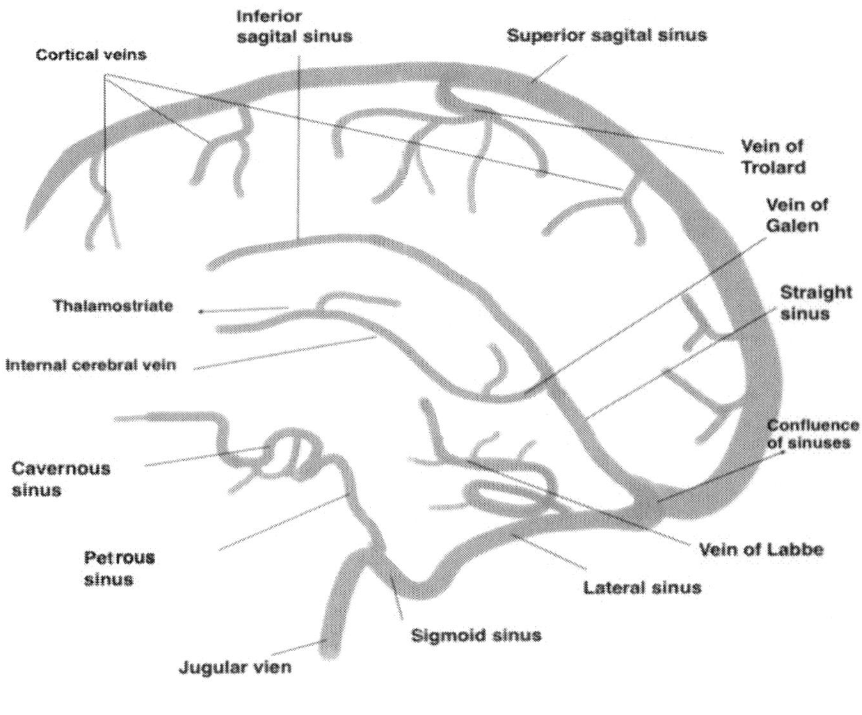

Figure 1.14. Superficial and deep venous system.

Deep venous drainage

The deep cerebral veins drain blood from the deep structures and join in a big central "vein of Galen "that in turn joins with the *inferior sagittal sinus* to form the *straight sinus*. The straight sinus then joins the superficial venous system to form the *confluence of sinuses*.

▪ Physiology of blood flow

Cerebral blood flow (CBF) is normally 50 to 54 ml/100 g/minute. CBF is tightly regulated based on the brain's needs. Autoregulation prevents excess amounts of blood (*hyperemia*) from harming the brain due to resultant increased intracranial pressure (ICP). Also, normal autoregulation prevents a drop in supply below 18 to 20 ml /100 g/ minute (the critical threshold). Neuronal dysfunction and untimely death or necrosis occurs if CBF drops below 8 to 10 ml/100g/minute. Understanding CBF physiology is very essential when treating patients with acute brain injuries secondary to shock, stroke, bleed, and traumatic brain injury.

Another important physiological parameter is cerebral perfusion pressure (CPP). CPP is calculated by subtracting intracranial pressure (ICP) from mean arterial pressure (MAP). Normal CPP is above 50 mmHg. Normal ICP is less than 15 mmHg. Due to autoregulation, cerebral blood vessels are able to change the flow by changing their diameter. When blood pressure increases, the intracranial arteries constrict and when it decreases, they dilatate to keep CBF within normal range. The changes mainly occur at the level of arterioles. Another factor that affects arterioles' diameter is carbon dioxide (high levels act as a vasodilator in the brain, and low levels constrict vessels). The change in vessel diameter affects blood flow by changing cerebrovascular resistance (CVR).

CBF is calculated by dividing CPP into CVR (CBF = CPP / CVR). CVR is determined by four major variables: metabolic control (or 'metabolic autoregulation'), mechanical autoregulation, chemical control (by arterial pCO_2 and pO_2) and neural control.

Another important fact when discussing CPP is that increased ICP does not decrease CPP solely by increasing counter pressure. It expresses more deleterious effect on CPP by also increased interstitial hydrostatic pressure and compressing intracranial arteries causing increased CVR.

References

1. *Neuromarketing: Applications, Challenges and Promises.* Solomon, Pravin Raj. 2, s.l. : Biomedical Journal of Scientific & Technical Research, 2018.
2. *Ischemic neuronal damage.* Taoufik E, Probert L. 2008, Curr Pharm Des, pp. 3565-73.
3. Brainstem -Neuroanatomy. [Online] Feb 17, 2014. http://pmcanatomy.blogspot.com/.
4. M. Leo Barahona, J. P. Mora Encinas , R. Querol Pascual , J. Structural and Functional anatomy of cerebellum. More than a motor conception. [Online] European Society of Radiology. www.myESR.org.

2

Types of Stroke and Pathophysiology

There are two types of stroke or "brain attack": *ischemic* where there is blockage (occlusion) of a blood vessel (cerebral artery) in the brain and *hemorrhagic* where there is leakage of blood from blood vessel into the brain tissue (intracerebral; ICH) or into the space between the skull and brain (subarachnoid; SAH).

▪ Ischemic stroke

Ischemic stroke is a heterogenous disease with many different causes, presentations, acute management and prevention. There are four main types of ischemic stroke: large vessel occlusion (LVO) stroke; small vessel (lacunar) stroke (SVS); global ischemia; and cerebral venous thrombosis (CVT). Ischemic stroke can also be categorized based on cause: atherosclerotic (30%); cardioembolic (20%); small vessel disease (15%); cryptogenic (30%), and rare causes (5%). In further discussion, we will focus on the four main types because it is more useful when managing ischemic stroke acutely (Figure 2.1).

Large vessel occlusion (LVO)

Large vessel occlusion usually causes strokes involving the cerebral cortex, where neurons reside. This makes LVO prognosis worse than small vessel type. Large vessel occlusion is the main focus in acute stroke management nowadays because it determines candidacy for the new innovative stroke treatment: endovascular treatment (EVT).

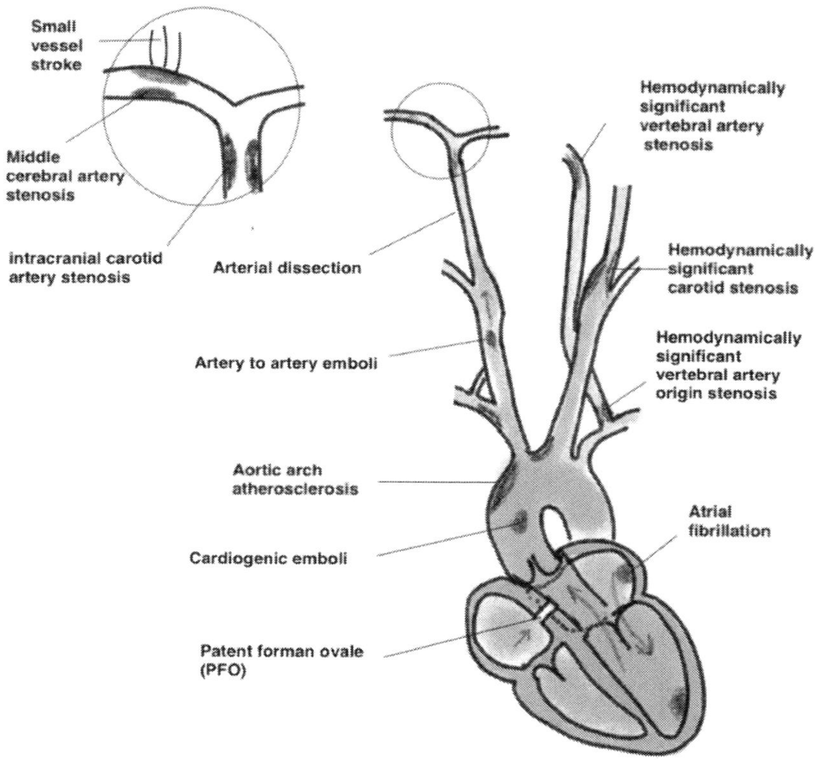

Figure 2.1. Different sources of ischemic stroke.

LVO can result from an embolus that dislodges in intracranial arteries after originating from the heart (commonly due to atrial fibrillation) or from more proximal area of the artery (commonly atherosclerotic plaque or arterial dissection). Sometimes the blockage is a result of local thrombotic event (commonly due to local atherosclerotic disease).

1. *Embolic stroke* usually presents with maximal neurological deficit quickly over seconds to minutes.
2. *Atherothrombotic* or atherosclerotic strokes usually reach maximal neurological deficit over minutes to hours. It is not uncommon in this type of stroke that patient symptoms fluctuate especially with blood pressure fluctuation.

Small vessel stroke (SVS)

Small vessel strokes typically affect the deeper portion of the brain which is made mainly of axons and glial cells. Small vessel strokes are usually the result of occlusion/collapse of very small vessels due to chronic injury secondary to uncontrolled hypertension (HTN) and diabetes mellitus (DM) and tobacco use. In this stroke type, the visible large blood vessels are not involved and thus EVT has no role in acute management of this type of stroke. Though it is possible to distinguish SVS from LVO strokes; however, this is not always easy and possible by providers who are not well trained with neurological examination. Chapter 3 will discuss in more detail how to distinguish LVO (cortical) stroke from SVS (lacunar) stroke.

Global ischemia or hypoxia

Global ischemic/hypoxemic strokes are not common, and they usually result from lack of nutrients (glucose mainly) and oxygen supply to the entire brain due to severe hypotension or hypoxia. This type will not be discussed extensively in this book due to lack of effective treatment to reverse symptoms and injury.

Cerebral Venous Thrombosis (CVT)

This type of venous stroke has different pathophysiology, presentation, and treatment compared to arterial strokes. Therefore, cerebral venous thrombosis will be discussed further in chapter 4.

Penumbra and collateral circulation in LVO stroke

The introduction of the concept of ischemic "*penumbra*" and its subsequent progression to completed stroke over time, led to a huge change from considering ischemic stroke as an irreversible catastrophe to treatable disease. The discovery of thrombolytic therapy and EVT is based on this concept and is considered one of the most important breakthrough discoveries in medicine in the last 25 years.

The penumbra is defined as the deprived (hypoperfused) area surrounding the ischemic dead area (core) in which blood flow is low to maintain electric activity but sufficient to preserve viability of the neurons (by preserving ion channels) (Figure 2.2). However, the penumbra is not static due to wave of deleterious metabolic cascade that spreads from the core to the surrounding tissue (excitotoxicity, oxidative stress, and inflammatory response). This leads to the expansion of the ischemic core with subsequent worsening clinical outcome [(1)].

The cerebral *collateral circulation* (CC) is what prolongs the life of ischemic tissues around the core in LVO strokes, so CC awareness and assessment is essential while managing LVO ischemic strokes (Figure 2.3).

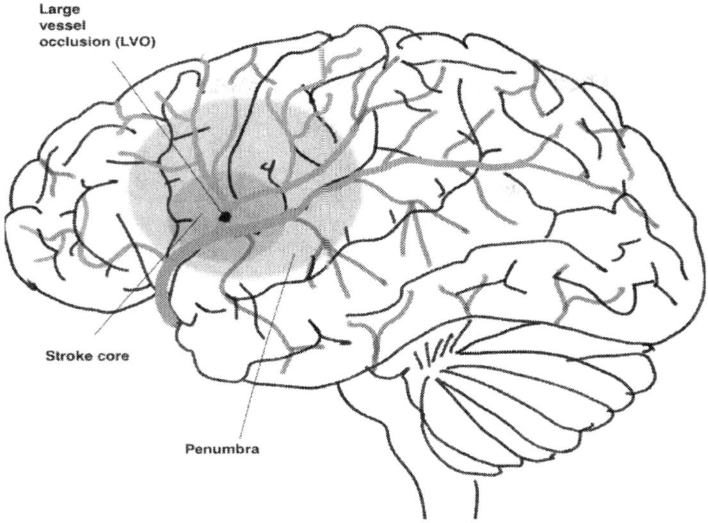

Figure 2.2. Large vessel occlusion with resultant progressive stroke. Stroke core contains dead brain tissue and penumbra zone contains dysfunctional (silent) neurons that are in process of slow death; if blood flow is not restored on timely fashion penumbra turns into core.

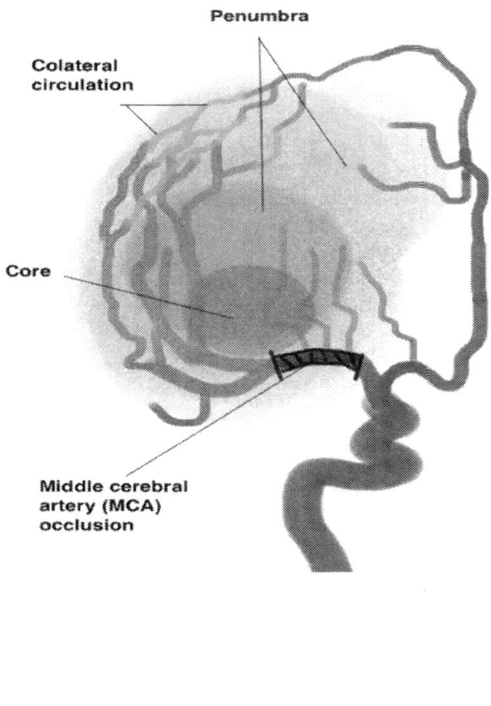

Figure 2.3. Penumbra is result of collateral circulation. The more robust collateral circulation, the more sustainable the penumbra.

CC is formed by network of vascular channels that maintain cerebral blood flow when main feeder vessels are blocked. The presence of penumbra is a result of good CC. However, not all patients with LVO stroke have the same ability to develop CC. Adequate CC may contribute to the maintenance of tissue viability in the absence of recanalization. Poor collaterals are demonstrated to be strong predictors of both response to EVT and functional outcome. There are specific measures that treating physicians should be aware of and consider in acute stroke to improve, or at least preserve, CC until more specific treatment is applied [(2)].

▪ Hemorrhagic stroke

Hemorrhagic stroke, like ischemic stroke, is also a heterogenous disease that varies in causes, presentations, acute management and prevention. There are four main categories for hemorrhagic stroke: intracerebral hemorrhage (ICH); subarachnoid hemorrhage (SAH); subdural hemorrhage (SDH); and epidural hemorrhage (EDH) (Figure 2.4).

Intracerebral hemorrhage (ICH)

Intracerebral hemorrhage (ICH) accounts for 8-13% of all strokes and results from a wide variety of disorders. It has higher chance to cause death or major disability than ischemic stroke or subarachnoid hemorrhage. Intracerebral hemorrhages and resultant edema can disrupt or compress adjacent brain tissue, leading to neurological dysfunction. If volume of hemorrhage is significant, it can cause displacement of brain parenchyma and possibly increased intracranial pressure (ICP) and potentially fatal herniation syndromes.

There are many causes for ICH; however, the most common cause is hypertension (HTN). Other causes include traumatic head injury, coagulopathy, cerebral amyloid angiopathy, intracranial neoplasm, arteriovenous malformation (common in younger patients), aneurysm rupture, (common in elderly), hemorrhagic transformation of an ischemic stroke, cerebral venous thrombosis, sympathomimetic drug abuse, Moya Moya disease, sickle cell disease, eclampsia or postpartum vasculopathy, infection and vasculitis.

Nontraumatic ICH most commonly results from hypertensive damage to blood vessel walls (eg, chronic hypertension, eclampsia, drug abuse). Chronic hypertension produces a small vessel vasculopathy characterized by lipohyalinosis, fibrinoid necrosis, and development of Charcot-Bouchard aneurysms, affecting penetrating arteries throughout the brain. The most common sites for ICH include the basal ganglia (40-50%), lobar regions (20-50%), thalamus (10-15%), pons (5-12%), cerebellum (5-10%), and other brainstem sites (1-5%) [3].

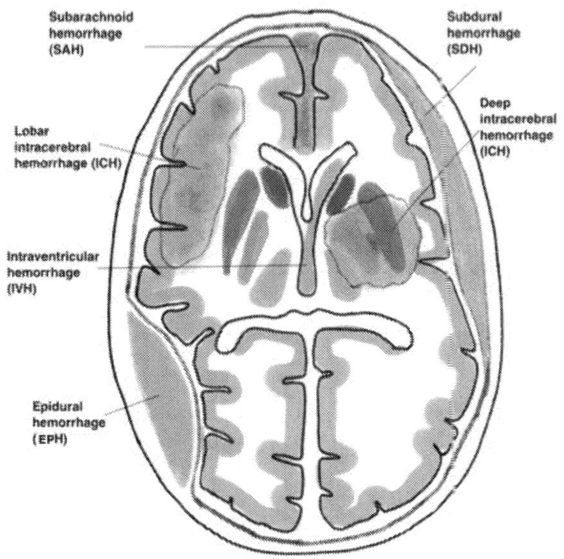

Figure 2.4. Different types of cranial bleed.

Table 2.1. ICH Scoring [4]

Component	ICH point
GCS score	
3-4	2
5-12	1
13-15	0
Volume, cm^3	
> 30	1
< 30	0
IVH	
Yes	1
No	0
Infratentorial origin of ICH	
Yes	1
No	0
Age, y	
> 80	1
< 80	0
Total ICH score	0-6

ICH scoring system

The ICH scoring system helps to determine severity and prognosis of ICH (Table 2.1). This score helps predict outcome at 30 days. The higher the score, the higher the probability of death [4]. The scoring system components are: GCS score on initial presentation (or after resuscitation); ICH volume, volume on initial CT calculated using ABC/2 method; and presence of any IVH on initial CT. Score 0 corresponds to 0% mortality; score 1, 13%; score 2, 26%; score 3, 72%, score 4, 97%, score 5 and 6, 100% mortality.

Complications of ICH

Hematoma expansion occurs in 30%. This leads to worse outcome. Risk factors are ICH volume, early presentation after symptom onset, anticoagulation, and spot sign on CT angiography [5].

Brain edema occurs in all cases due to inflammation and coagulation response after ICH. This leads to worse outcome [6].

Hydrocephalus occurs due to associated IVH. This leads to worse outcome [4].

Seizures occur mainly with cortical involvement. Delayed seizures are associated with worse functional outcome [7] [8].

Intraventricular hemorrhage (IVH)

Intraventricular hemorrhage is either an extension from intracerebral hemorrhage (thalamic bleed) into the ventricular space or a primary intraventricular hemorrhage that frequently arises from subependymal structures including the germinal matrix, AVMs, or cavernous angiomas [3].

Subarachnoid hemorrhage (SAH)

Subarachnoid hemorrhage (SAH) is bleeding from intracranial vessels (usually aneurysm or vascular malformation) into the subarachnoid space between the pial and arachnoid membranes. The most common cause for SAH is traumatic head injury. However, the focus in this book is on aneurysmal or vascular SAH.

When an aneurysm ruptures, it releases blood under high arterial pressure into the subarachnoid space. This allows blood to spread around the brain and spinal cord with CSF. This directly damages local tissues, increasing intracranial pressure (ICP) and irritating meningeal tissue.

Complications of SAH

Re-bleed occurs in ~ 7% of patients (mainly in first 24-48 hours) and is associated with a dismal outcome. The mortality rate is 80%. Re-bleed rate is less with good clinical grades (Grades 1 to 3, Hunt Grades I and II) than in poor clinical grades (Grades 4 to 9, Hunt Grades III to V) [(9) (10)].

Hydrocephalus occurs in 20% to 30% of patients. Onset can be acute, within 48 hours after SAH, or rarely chronic, weeks and even months after the SAH [(11)].

Delayed cerebral ischemia (DCI) is very common (symptomatic in 16%, asymptomatic in 21%) and it worsens outcome [(12)].

Low sodium level (hyponatremia) occurs in 50% of SAH patients. SIADH is the most frequent cause followed by cerebral salt wasting (CSW) [(13)].

Cardiac manifestations such as ECG changes and low systolic cardiac function are not uncommon in SAH patients.

Seizures occur in 3% to 26%. Late or recurrent epilepsy occurs in 7% to 12% [(14)]. More details are discussed in chapter 13.

Table 2.2. SAH clinical grading systems.

Grade	Botterell et al.	Hunt and Hess	WFNS
1	Conscious with or without signs of blood in the subarachnoid space	Asymptomatic or minimal headache and slight nuchal rigidity	GCS 15, no motor deficit
2	Drowsy without significant neurological deficit	Moderate-to-severe headache nuchal rigidity, no neurological deficit other than cranial nerve palsy	GCS 13 to 14, no motor deficit
3	Drowsy with neurological deficit and probably intracerebral clot	Drowsy, confusion, or mild focal deficit	GCS 13 to 14, with motor deficit
4	Major neurological deficit, deteriorating because of large intracerebral clots or neurological deficit but pre-existing cerebrovascular disease	Stupor, moderate-to-severe hemiparesis, possibly early decerebrate rigidity and without motor deficit older patients with less severe vegetative disturbances	GCS 7 to 12, with or without motor deficit
5	Moribund or near moribund with failing vital centers and extensor rigidity	Deep coma, decerebrate rigidity, moribund appearance	GCS 3 to 6, with or without motor deficit

SAH grading system

There are many clinical and radiographic scoring systems for subarachnoid hemorrhage (SAH) to grade degree and prognosis such as Hunt and Hess Scale, Fisher Scale, Glasgow Coma Score (GCS), and World Federation of Neurological Surgeons Scale (WFNS) [15] (Tables 2.2, 2.3, 2.4).

Table 2.3. Fisher scale.

Fisher scale	
Grade	***CT Scan***
1	No blood visualized
2	A diffuse deposition of thin layer with all vertical layers of blood (interhemispheric fissure, insular cistern, ambient cistern) less than 1 mm thick
3	Localized clots and/or vertical layers of blood 1 mm or greater in thickness
4	Diffuse or no subarachnoid blood, but with intracerebral or intraventricular clots

Table 2.4. Glasgow Coma Scale (GCS).

GCS	
Parameter	**Score**
Eyes	
Open spontaneously	4
Open to verbal command	3
Open to pain	2
No eye opening	1
Best motor response	
Obeys to verbal command	6
Localizes to painful stimulus	5
Flexion withdrawal to pain	4
Abnormal flexion (decorticate rigidity) to pain	3
Abnormal extension (decerebrate rigidity) to pain	2
No response	1
Best verbal response	
Oriented and converses	5
Disoriented and converses	4
Inappropriate words	3
Incomprehensible sounds	2
No response	1

Brain aneurysms

The prevalence of unruptured intracranial aneurysms (UIAs) is around 3%, with 20–30% of patients harboring more than one aneurysm. UIAs can remain clinically silent, become symptomatic due to local mass effect or seizures, or progress towards rupture. SAH due to a ruptured aneurysm mortality rate is 25–50%.

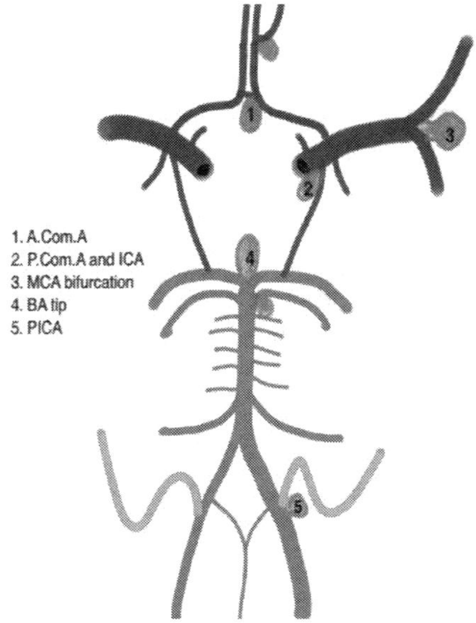

Figure 2.5. Most common locations of cerebral aneurysms by order 1 to 5.

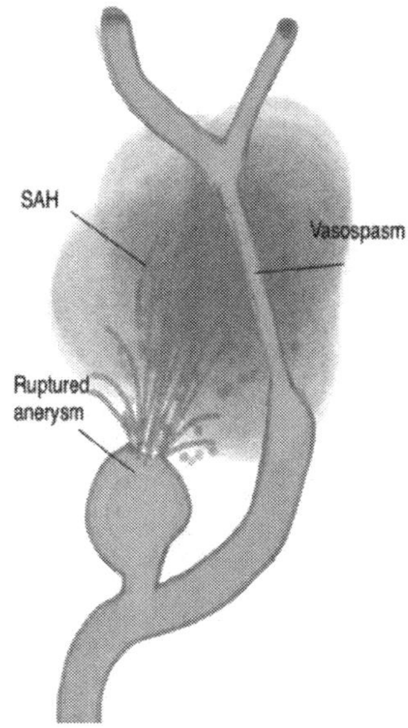

Figure 2.6. Aneurysm rupture and vasospasm.

Current hypotheses suggest the following mechanisms for aneurysm formation. There is initial apoptosis in vascular smooth muscle cells within the internal elastic lamina and collagen and/or elastin degradation. This is followed by remodeling process to strengthen the aneurysmal area. However, this might not result in stabilization and can lead to progression or even rupture under hemodynamic stress such as hypertension or nicotine consumption.

The probability of rupture is related to the tension on the aneurysm wall (law of La Place; that is related to radius and pressure gradient). This explains why larger aneurysm are at higher risk of rupture (≤5 mm, 2%; 6-10 mm, 40%) [16] (Table 15.1). More details about risk factors and clinical presentation are discussed in chapters 14 and 15.

Table 2.5. Risk factors for aneurysms.

Risk factors for developing aneurysms
Non-modifiable
Genetic disorders that weaken arteries Polycystic kidney disease Arteriovenous malformations History of aneurysm in a first-degree family member Age over 40
Modifiable
Uncontrolled hypertension Smoking Drug abuse (cocaine or amphetamines Intravenous drug abuse (mycotic aneurysms due to infection)

Table 2.6. PHASES Risk Score.

PHASES Aneurysm Risk Score	
Criteria	Points
Population	
North American, European (not Finnish)	0
Japanese	3
Finnish	5
Hypertension	
No	0
Yes	1
Age	
< 70	0
≥ 70 y	1
Size of aneurysm	
< 7.0 mm	0
7-9.9 mm	3
10-19.9 mm	6
≥ 20.0 mm	10
Earlier SAH from different aneurysm	
No	0
Yes	1
Site of aneurysm	
ICA	0
MCA	2
ACA or posterior circulation	4

There are many risk factors that promote aneurysm formation (Table 2.5 and 2.6) [17].

There are several traditional factors for aneurysm rupture including: hypertension, smoking, size, location, growth, family history and multiple aneurysms with history of rupture (greatest risk factor). In addition to these traditional risks factors, there are other risks factors summarized in PHASES score (Table 2.6) that was developed as a practical risk score to predict a patient's 5-year risk of aneurysm rupture rate (≤ 2, 0.4%; 3, 0.7%; 4, 0.9%; 5, 1.7%; 7,2.4%; 8,3.2%; 9,4.3%; 10, 5.3%; 11, 7.2%; ≥12,17.8%) [17].

Brain arteriovenous malformations (AVMs)

Brain AVM consists of an abnormal tangle of blood vessels that allows an artery to connect directly to a vein therefore bypassing capillaries and brain tissue (Figure 2.7). Brain AVMs are much less common (< 1% in population) than cerebral aneurysm. AVMs can manifest with bleeding (most common presentation, 70%; ICH, SAH, IVH), seizures, and other neurologic issues (such as weakness and numbness). However, unruptured AVMs are often asymptomatic and only discovered accidentally on imaging. Bleeding is associated with a 10-20% mortality and a 10-20% disability.

The bleed from AVM can lead to similar complications related to ICH, IVH or SAH based on the type of bleed they cause. Spetzler Martin *Grading* Scale (Table 2.7) is used to assess variable risks from surgical treatment. This scale estimates the risk of open neurosurgery for a patient with AVM based on size, pattern of venous drainage, and eloquence of brain location [18].

AVM rupture risk factors are not well established; however, a history of hemorrhage, deep AVM location, deep venous drainage and the presence of associated aneurysms are likely factors that increase the risk of hemorrhage [19] .

Treatment decisions (treat or not treat, modality of treatment [open surgical, EVT, radiosurgery]) of brain AVM is not straightforward and very complex for this book to discuss. In an effort to stratify brain AVM based on need for treatment, an NIH-funded study (ARUBA) was conducted. This study advocates conservative approach to unruptured AVMs in the short-term; however, the management implications have been widely debated since the natural history of AVMs in the medically treated arm was not negligible (>3% rupture risk per year) and a longer-term study follow-up is pending [20].

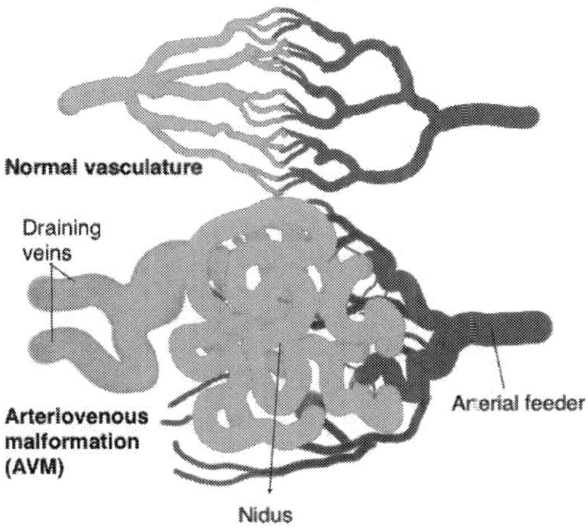

Figure 2.7. Normal vessels versus AVM.

Table 2.7. AVM Spetzler Martin Grading Scale

Spetzler Martin **Grading *Scale***	
Feature	**Points**
Size of AVM	
Small (<3 cm)	1
Medium (3-6 cm)	2
Large > 6	3
Eloquence of adjacent brain	
Non-eloquent	0
Eloquent	1
Pattern of venous drainage	
Superficial	0
Deep	1

Subdural hemorrhage (SDH)

Subdural hematoma (SDH) is a result of bleeding from bridging veins within the subdural space in between the inner layer of the dura and external layer that is attached to skull. It usually results from high-speed impact to the skull. Bridging veins can bleed easily if they are already stretched due to brain atrophy in elderly. Older age and anticoagulation are at highest risk even with less severe head injuries. SDH may also be spontaneous or due to procedure (lumbar puncture). Rates of mortality and morbidity can be high, even with the best medical and neurosurgical care [21].

SDH is usually characterized based on size, location and acuity (acute: < 3 days; subacute: 3-7 days; chronic: weeks; very often mixed). The neurological condition of the patient also determines outcome and treatment options. Acute SDH frequently causes coma on admission due to tremendous mass effect. For less dramatic cases, simple classification of mild (GCS 9-13) and moderate (14-15) is frequently used. In acute SDH, patients are likely to have lucid interval then deteriorate. Timely treatment (medical and surgical) before further decline is essential [21].

Epidural hemorrhage (EDH)

EDH is bleeding into the space between dura and bone of skull or spine. It usually results from a brief linear contact force to the skull that causes separation of the periosteal dura from bone and disruption of interposed vessels (arteries or veins) due to shearing stress. Extension of EDH usually is limited by suture lines owing to the tight attachment of the dura at these locations. It occurs in 2% of patients with head injuries and 5–15% of patients with fatal head injuries. It is associated with skull fractures in 85–95%. It is considered the most serious complication of head injury, requiring immediate diagnosis and surgical intervention. Intracranial epidural hematoma may be acute (58%), subacute (31%), or chronic (11%). Mortality rate 5–50% [22].

EDH is most commonly located in temporoparietal region and the middle meningeal artery (66%) and less commonly in anterior ethmoidal artery (due to frontal injury), transverse or sigmoid sinus (due to occipital injury), and superior sagittal sinus (due to vertex injury) [22].

Spinal epidural hematoma (SEDH) may be spontaneous or may follow minor trauma, such as lumbar puncture or epidural anesthesia. Spontaneous SEDH may be associated with anticoagulation, thrombolysis, blood dyscrasias, coagulopathies, thrombocytopenia, neoplasms, or vascular malformations. The peridural venous plexus usually is involved, though arterial sources of hemorrhage also occur. The dorsal aspect of the thoracic or lumbar region is involved most commonly, with expansion limited to a few vertebral levels [22].

References:

1. Ramos-Cabrer, Pedro. Targeting the Ischemic Penumbra. [Online] Dec 16, 2010. https://www.ahajournals.org/doi/10.1161/STROKEAHA.110.596684.
2. Bang, Oh Young. Collateral Circulation in Ischemic Stroke: Assessment Tools and Therapeutic Strategies. [Online] Nov 2015. https://www.ncbi.nlm.nih.gov/pmc/articles/PMC4624512/.
3. Liebeskind, David S. Intracranial Hemorrhage. [Online] Dec 7, 2018. https://emedicine.medscape.com/article/1163977-overview.
4. *The ICH Score A Simple, Reliable Grading Scale for Intracerebral Hemorrhage.* Hemphill, J. Claude. 2001, Stroke, pp. 891-897.
5. *Hematoma Expansion Following Acute Intracerebral Hemorrhage.* H. Bart Brouwers, MD. 2013, Cerebrovasc Dis, pp. 195-201.
6. H, Zheng. Mechanism and Therapy of Brain Edema after Intracerebral Hemorrhage. [Online] Apr 26, 2016. https://www.ncbi.nlm.nih.gov/pubmed/27110940.
7. Kwang-Moo Woo, M.D., Seung-Yeob Yang, M.D. and Keun-Tae Cho, M.D. [Online] Oct 2012. https://www.ncbi.nlm.nih.gov/pmc/articles/PMC3488638/.
8. Biffi, Alessandro, Rattani, Abbas and Anderson, Christopher D. [Online] Oct 2016. https://www.ncbi.nlm.nih.gov/pmc/articles/PMC5035821/.
9. *The risk of rebleeding from ruptured intracranial aneurysms.* Rosenørn J, Eskesen V, Schmidt K. 67, s.l. : J Neurosurg, 1987.
10. *Predictors and Impact of Aneurysm Rebleeding After Subarachnoid Hemorrhage.* Andrew M. Naidech, MD, MSPH, Nazli Janjua, MD and Kurt T. Kreiter, PhD. 3, s.l. : JAMA Neurology, 2005.
11. *Hydrocephalus After Aneurysmal Subarachnoid Hemorrhage.* Anand V. Germanwala, MD'Correspondence information about the author MD Anand V. GermanwalaEmail the author MD Anand V. Germanwala , Judy Huang, MD , Rafael J. Tamargo, MD. 2, s.l. : Neurosurgery Clinics, 2010, Vol. 21.
12. *Defining Vasospasm After Subarachnoid Hemorrhage.* Jennifer A. Frontera, Andres Fernandez , J. Michael Schmidt ,. 6, s.l. : Stroke, 2009, Vol. 40.
13. *Diagnosis and Management of Hyponatremia in Patients with Aneurysmal Subarachnoid Hemorrhage.* Mittal, Neena I. Marupudi and Sandeep. 4, s.l. : J Clin Med, 2015, Vol. 4.
14. *Seizures and Epilepsy following Aneurysmal Subarachnoid Hemorrhage : Incidence and Risk Factors.* Kyu-Sun Choi, M.D., Hyoung-Joon Chun, M.D., Hyeong-Joong Yi, M.D. 2, s.l. : J Korean Neurosurg Soc, 2009, Vol. 46.
15. *110Review ArticleAbstractNumerous systems are reported for grading the clinical condition of patients followingsubarachnoid hemorrhage (SAH). The literature was reviewed for articles pertaining tothe grading of such patients, including publications on the.* Macdonald, David S. Rosen and R. Loch. s.l. : Neurocritical Care, 2005, Vol. 2.
16. *Cerebral aneurysms: Formation, progression and developmental chronology.* Nima Etminan, M.D., Bruce A. Buchholz, Ph.D., Rita Dreier, Ph.D. 2, s.l. : Transl Stroke Res., 2013, Vol. 5.
17. Dr Jacoba P Greving, PhD Marieke J H Wermer, MD Prof Robert D Brown Jr, MD. Development of the PHASES score for prediction of risk of rupture of intracranial aneurysms: a pooled analysis of six prospective cohort studies. [Online] Nov 27, 2013. https://www.thelancet.com/journals/laneur/article/PIIS1474-4422(13)70263-1/fulltext.

18. *Validation of the Supplemented Spetzler-Martin Grading System for Brain Arteriovenous Malformations in a Multicenter Cohort of 1009 Surgical Patients.* Helen Kim, PhD, Adib A. Abla, MD, Jeffrey Nelson, MS. 1, s.l. : Neurosurgery, 2016, Vol. 76.
19. *Hemorrhage Rates and Risk Factors in the Natural History Course of Brain Arteriovenous Malformations.* W. Caleb Rutledge, Nerissa U. Ko, Michael T. Lawton. 5, s.l. : Transl Stroke Res, 2014, Vol. 5.
20. *Medical management with or without interventional therapy for unruptured brain arteriovenous malformations (ARUBA): a multicentre, non-blinded, randomised trial.* Prof J P Mohr, MD * Prof Michael K Parides, PhD Prof Christian Stapf, MD. 9917, s.l. : The Lancet, 2014, Vol. 383.
21. Richard J Meagher, MD and Chief Editor: Helmi L Lutsep, MD. Subdural Hematoma. [Online] July 26, 2018. https://emedicine.medscape.com/article/1137207-overview.
22. Khairat, Ali and Waseem, Muhammad. Epidural Hematoma. [Online] Nov 15, 2018. https://www.ncbi.nlm.nih.gov/books/NBK518982/.
23. Tibor Becske, MD. [Online] Dec 2018. https://emedicine.medscape.com/article/1164341-overview#a4.

3

Ischemic Stroke Syndromes, Mimics, Chameleons

Ischemic stroke can affect cerebral cortex (frontal, parietal, temporal and occipital lobes); subcortical area (internal capsule, thalamus, basal ganglia); brainstem; or cerebellum. This classification is very helpful clinically because the etiology and clinical management of the different types, especially cortical and subcortical strokes, is different. For instance, a middle cerebral artery occlusion resulting in a cortical stroke usually results from an embolus from either the heart, aortic arch or carotid artery, whereas a tiny infarct in the internal capsule is usually due to blockage of small penetrating artery (lacunar infarct). An embolic cortical stroke causing large vessel occlusion (LVO) might benefit from advanced endovascular treatment (EVT) while lacunar stroke does not.

▪ Cortical stroke

Cortical strokes usually affect higher cognitive function. Depending on the side of the brain and the lobe involved, different functions are impaired (Table 3.1 and Figure 3.1). The distribution of the cortical sensory or motor deficits follows the "homunculus" of the cortex. For example, a left middle cerebral artery stroke to the inferior frontal lobe may result in an expressive aphasia, an inability to express language. A dominant posterior cerebral artery stroke may result in pure alexia, a disturbance of reading. Dominant cortical strokes lead to agraphia, an inability to write, and acalculia, a disturbance of calculation. Right parietal strokes may result in a neglect syndrome, a denial of deficits and stimuli on the contralateral body, or difficulty in spatial organization which results in impaired drawing, copying or interpreting pictures. It is rare for a subcortical stroke to disrupt these higher order mental functions (1) (2).

In cortical strokes, there is preferential involvement of different motor areas. For example, a left MCA stroke will often result in a motor deficit involving the right face and arm more than leg, while a left ACA stroke will affect the right leg more than face and arm. Focal weakness of a distal extremity may occur as well. In contrast, a subcortical stroke presentation may involve face, arm and leg to an equal extent. This is based on the close proximity of corticospinal tract fibers to each other as they run through the subcortical structures such as the internal capsule and brainstem. The same concept applies on sensory loss in cortical stroke. Thus, it would be unusual for a cortical stroke to involve the entire contralateral hemibody. However, it is not uncommon for a small subcortical thalamic infarct to result in hemisensory face, arm and leg impairment [(2)].

The type of sensory loss in cortical stroke may present differently from subcortical sensory impairment. More specifically, a cortical stroke may result in loss of higher order sensory function. For example, with a parietal stroke, the patient may have contralateral agraphesthesia (loss of the ability to recognize a number or letter traced on a limb) and astereognosia (loss of ability to recognize objects by touch) despite intact primary sensory sensation [(2)].

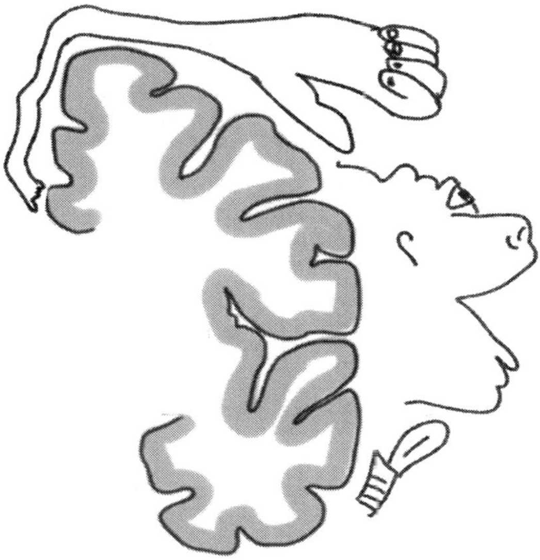

Figure 3.1. Brain homunculus. Face, language and hand have large representation areas as opposed to leg and toes.

Cortical stroke may result in visual disturbances. For example, occipital lobe infarcts will result in disturbance of vision in the contralateral visual field. Similar deficits can occur with cortical strokes affecting the temporal and parietal lobes where the optic radiations travel. It is rare for a subcortical stroke to impair vision [(2)].

Cortical stroke may present with a gaze deviation to the side of the stroke. This occurs when the frontal eye fields, responsible for horizontal gaze, are infarcted [(2)].

▪ Subcortical stroke

Subcortical strokes do not involve the cortex and are not usually associated with large vessel occlusion (Table 3.2).

Table 3.1. Cortical stroke syndromes.

Cortical stroke syndromes	
Anterior circulation strokes	
Left MCA syndrome Anterior (superior) division Posterior (inferior) division	-Sensorimotor loss in right face and arm, leg to a lesser extent. -Deviation of head/eyes toward the stroke. -Initial global aphasia then expressive aphasia. -Superior quadrantanopia/homonymous hemianopia. -Receptive aphasia.
Right MCA syndrome Anterior division Posterior division	-Sensorimotor loss in left face and arm, leg to a lesser extent. Ipsilateral deviation of head/eyes. -No impairment of alertness. -Superior quadrantanopia/homonymous hemianopia and left sided visual neglect
Left or right ACA syndrome	-Contralateral sensorimotor deficits involving the leg and sparing face and hand
Bilateral ACAs syndrome	-Paraplegia, incontinence, abulia and motor aphasia, personality changes, grasp reflex
AChA syndromes	Contralateral hemiplegia and hemi-hypoesthesia, homonymous hemianopsia
Left or right PCA syndrome PCA is a branch of basilar artery; however, it supplies structure that are supratentorial	-Contralateral homonymous hemianopia, paresthesias, and weakness. -Confusion, dizziness, nausea, memory loss, language dysfunction
Posterior circulation strokes	
Basilar artery (BA) stroke	-Vertigo, nausea and vomiting, headache, decreased level of consciousness, nystagmus, lateral gaze abnormalities, diplopia, pupillary changes, "locked in syndrome" in extreme cases
Posterior Inferior Cerebellar Stroke (PICA) (most common brainstem stroke)	-Lateral medullary syndrome, or "Wallenberg's syndrome". Vertigo, ipsilateral hemiataxia, dysarthria. Horner's syndrome (unilateral ptosis, miosis and facial anhidrosis).
Anterior Inferior Cerebellar Stroke (AICA)	-Vertigo and vomiting, nystagmus, dysarthria, falling to the side of the lesion, ipsilateral hemiataxia, loss of all modalities of sensation of the face, Ipsilateral facial paralysis, and hearing loss and tinnitus
Superior cerebellar stroke (SCA)	-Non-specific symptoms such as nausea/vomiting, headache and dizziness, Horner's syndrome

Table 3.2. Subcortical stroke syndromes.

Clinical Syndrome	Clinical findings	Stroke location
Pure motor hemiparesis (33-50%)	Contralateral motor deficit in face, arm, and leg	Posterior limb of the internal capsule corona radiata, or basis pontis
Pure sensory	Contralateral transient/persistent numbness, paresthesia and hemisensory deficit involving the face, arm, trunk and leg	Ventroposteriolateral nucleus of the thalamus or corona radiata
Ataxic-hemiparesis	Contralateral weakness that is more prominent in the leg, along with ipsilateral arm and leg incoordination	Posterior limb of the internal capsule, corona radiata or pons
Sensorimotor	Contralateral motor and sensory deficit in face, arm and leg	Thalamus, internal capsule or putamen-capsule-caudate
Dysarthria-clumsy hand syndrome	Dysarthria, dysphagia, Contralateral facial paresis and tongue weakness, Contralateral paresis/clumsiness of the arm and hand.	Basis pontis or internal capsule
Multiple subcortical infarcts and dementia	Dementia syndrome in addition to poor execution and motor programing, pseudobulbar effect, and parkinsonism	Caudate nucleus, globus pallidus, thalamus. Connecting fibers of frontal subcortical circuits

▪ Brainstem and cerebellar stroke

Table 3.3. Brainstem syndromes.

Syndrome	Anatomy	Clinical presentation
The midbrain Weber syndrome	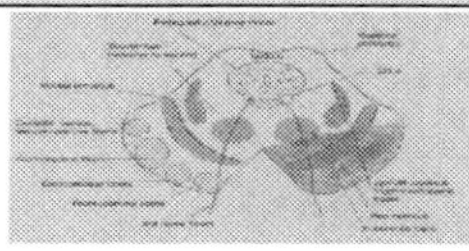	Contralateral hemiparesis Contralateral lower facial and tongue weakness Ipsilateral oculomotor nerve palsy
Benedickt syndrome	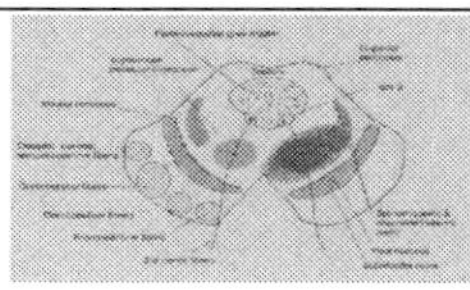	Contralateral hemiparesis Ipsilateral oculomotor nerve palsy Cerebellar ataxia Tremor and involuntary choreoathetotic movements
Claude's syndrome	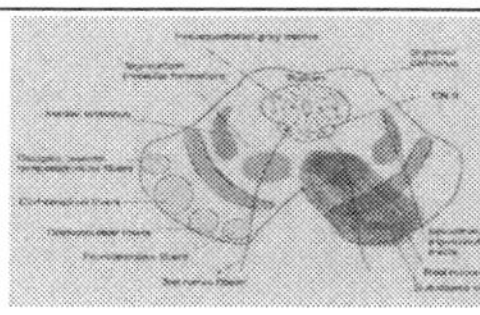	Contralateral hemiparesis Contralateral ataxia Ipsilateral oculomotor nerve palsy Tremor and involuntary choreoathetotic movements Contralateral hemiplegia of face, tongue, & shoulder
Medial pontine (Foville's) syndromes	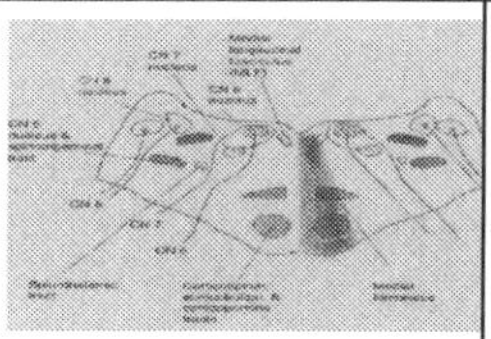	Contralateral hemiparesis and hemisensory loss Ipsilateral horizontal gaze palsy Internuclear ophthalmoplegia Ipsilateral facial nerve palsy
Lateral pontine (Marie-Foix) syndrome	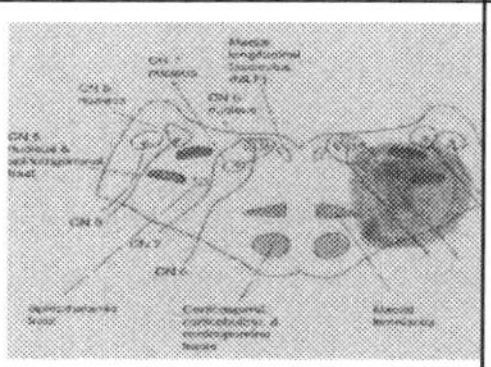	Contralateral loss of pain and temperature Ipsilateral paralysis of the upper and lower face Ipsilateral loss of lacrimation and reduced salivation Ipsilateral loss of taste from the anterior two-thirds of the tongue Loss of corneal reflex Ipsilateral facial hemianesthesia Nystagmus, nausea, vomiting, and vertigo Ipsilateral limb and gait ataxia Ipsilateral Horner's syndrome

Medial Medullary syndrome	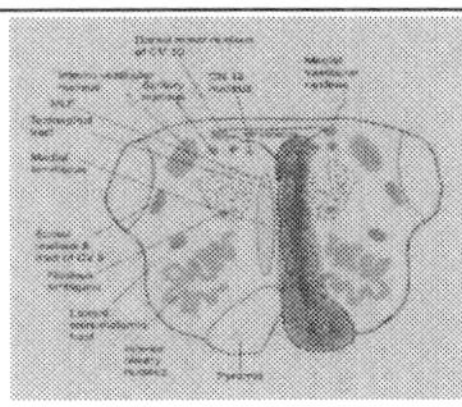	Deviation of the tongue to the side of the infarct on attempted protrusion Contralateral hemiparesis Contralateral loss of discriminative touch, conscious proprioception, and vibration sense
Lateral Medullary (Wallenberg) syndrome	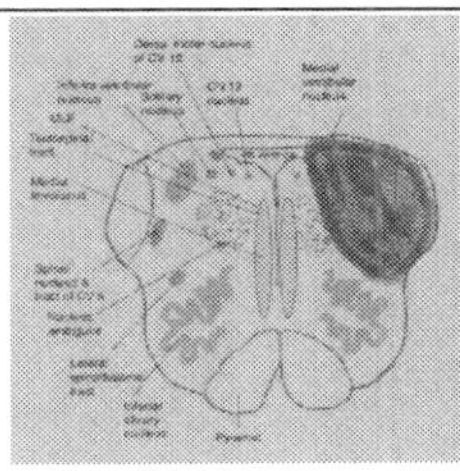	Contralateral body loss of pain and temperature Ipsilateral body loss of pain and temperature Ipsilateral laryngeal, pharyngeal, and palatal hemiparalysis Ipsilateral Horner's syndrome Nystagmus, nausea, vomiting, and vertigo Ipsilateral limb and gait ataxia Palatal myoclonus

Lesions which are subcortical in the brainstem may present with signs and symptoms such as extraocular movement impairments, diplopia, dysphagia, dysarthria, nystagmus. A subcortical stroke in the cerebellum may present with nausea, vomiting, vertigo, and imbalance. Exam may reveal nystagmus, ataxia and tremor [2]. Table 3.3 lists a comprehensive list of brainstem syndromes.

▪ Transient ischemic attack (TIA) and fluctuating stroke

TIAs result from temporary reduction or cessation of cerebral blood flow into a specific neurovascular distribution and clinical presentation similar to ischemic stroke based on the vessel involved and the cerebral territory it supplies. The AHA-endorsed definition of TIA is a transient episode of neurological dysfunction caused by focal brain, spinal cord, or retinal ischemia, without acute infarction on imaging. Unfortunately, there is no reliable method to stratify the risk of stroke after TIA. Thus, the author recommends that close observation during hospitalization has the potential to allow more rapid and frequent administration of tissue plasminogen activator should a stroke occur.

Obtaining STAT MRI and vascular images has been used frequently to distinguish TIA and fluctuating ischemic neurological deficit (FIND) from stroke and to stratify risk of recurrent symptoms to allow appropriate emergent management plan as mentioned in Table 3.4.

There are 200,000 to 500,000 TIAs diagnosed every year (0.3 % of ED visits). TIA carries a particularly high short-term risk of stroke, and approximately 15% of diagnosed strokes are preceded by TIAs. The risk of stroke after TIA is 11% at 7 days. The probability of stroke in the 5 years following a TIA is reported to be 24-29% [(3)]. This is why TIA deserves the same urgency in diagnosis and treatment and thus clinicians should have low threshold to make the initial diagnosis of TIA.

TIA is a very broad diagnosis that can be further classified based on presentation and etiology (Table 3.4). The author found the proposed FIND classification helpful with directing work up and treatment to a more specific root cause. This helps in implementing a more appropriate therapeutic approach based on the most likely etiology. This table summarizes different types of TIA based on presentation, etiology, work up and most appropriate therapeutic approach [(2)].

Table 3.4. Classification of fluctuating ischemic neurological deficit (FIND).

FIND	Presentation	Etiology	Urgent work up	Treatment
Resolving-Cortical (RC)	- Similar to any of the cortical syndromes described earlier in this chapter	-Cardio-embolic or artery to artery (not hemodynamically significant stenosis) embolus that resolves spontaneously due to intrinsic thrombolytic system -Symptoms could resolve also due to development of cortical collateral circulation (CCC)	-Head Non-contrast (NCCT) -Head & Neck CT Angiogram (H&N CTA) -MRI (to reset IV tPA time window) -Coagulation panel if AFib	-Intravenous fluid (IVF) for hydration -Optimize anticoagulation (AC) immediately if Afib -Dual anti-platelet (DAP) immediately if artery to artery embolus
Hemodynamic-Atherosclerotic (HA)	-Similar to cortical syndromes described earlier -There is often long history of fluctuation over many days or weeks -Usually very high BP	-Decreased blood flow due to hemodynamically significant stenosis (due to atherosclerosis or dissection) in cervical or intracranial arterial system; might be also associated with artery to artery embolus that resolve due to intrinsic thrombolytic system -Symptoms could resolve due to development of CCC	-Head NCCT -H&N CTA -MRI (to reset IV tPA time window) -Coagulation panel if associated with Afib	-IV fluid for hydration -DAP immediately -Determine & attain ideal SBP based on fluctuation (usually 140-180; in more critical stenosis up to 220)
Suturing-Small Vessel (SSV)	-Similar to any of the subcortical syndromes described earlier in this chapter	-The cause of fluctuation/deterioratio n is uncertain -No strong clinical and imaging predictors are established	-Head NCCT -H&N CTA -MRI (to reset IV tPA time window) -Lacunar infarcts may be associated with higher BP compared to non-lacunar infarcts	-IV fluid for hydration -DAP immediately No specific BP criteria needed -HTN in acute phase is not proven to be harmful but is considered as a risk factor

▪ Stroke mimics

Stroke mimics commonly confound the diagnosis of stroke. One study reported that 19% of patients diagnosed with acute ischemic stroke by neurologists before NCCT actually had non-cerebrovascular causes for their symptoms. Mimics cannot always be ruled out in the ED. Thrombolysis is usually well tolerated in mimics. Therefore, clinicians should not spend much time on all patients to improve diagnostic accuracy, knowing that time lost is harmful and will only prevent treating one mimic out of 100 patients. The most frequent stroke mimics include the following [(4)]: Seizure (17%), systemic infection (17%), brain tumor (15%), toxic-metabolic disorders, such as hyponatremia and hypoglycemia (13%), positional vertigo (6%), and conversion disorder.

There have been multiple attempts to develop a scoring system to help distinguish real strokes from mimics. Table 3.5 explains a scoring method called FABS. FABS includes six variables: absence of facial droop, negative history of atrial fibrillation, age, systolic blood pressure at presentation, history of seizures, and isolated sensory deficit without limb weakness at presentation. A score of 3 points or more identifies patients with stroke mimics (sensitivity, 90%; specificity, 91%; Table 3.5).

Another proposed scoring method is Tele Stroke Mimic Score (TSMS), with variables such as age, medical history (atrial fibrillation, hypertension, and convulsion), facial paralysis, and NIHSS score ≤14 as independent factors of stroke mimics. Because FABS and the Tele Stroke Mimic Score can be used with simple examination and vital signs, patients can be evaluated in a short time even in a busy ED, and the necessity of carrying out head MRI can be judged from the scoring result [(5)]. In the prehospital and ED settings, hypoglycemia is a common stroke mimic and is particularly important to consider, since it can be readily detected and corrected.

Table 3.5 FABS Scoring System.

FABS Scoring System [5]		
Clinical feature	**Sensitivity** %	**Specificity** %
Absence of facial droop	94	71
Age < 50	53	86
Absence of Afib	73	74
Presence of isolated sensory deficit	15	97
History of seizure	14	97
FABS ≥3 could identify mimics with 90% sensitivity and 91 % specificity		

Table 3.6. Examples of Chameleons.

Examples of Chameleons [7]	
Stroke	**Presentation**
Bilateral thalamic stoke	Persistent acute global amnesia
Critical carotid stenosis	Glioma (in watershed areas)
Limb shaking TIA	Focal epilepsy
Cortical stroke	Peripheral nerve lesion
Bilateral occipital strokes	Confusion/delirium

Stroke chameleons

Stroke chameleons (Table 3.6) are ischemic strokes that present similar to non–stroke conditions. They may interfere with prompt recognition and treatment of stroke. Stroke chameleons may result in patients not receiving appropriate care. Consideration of key discriminating features of stroke mimics and chameleons can assist clinicians in proper triaging of suspected strokes [6]. The most likely chameleons are altered mental status (AMS), syncope, hypertensive emergency, systemic infection, and suspected acute coronary syndrome (ACS). Patients diagnosed with hypertensive emergency or AMS have an 8% and 7% chance of having an acute stroke. Physicians should consider stroke in patients with these diagnoses and have a lower threshold to obtain neuroimaging with subsequent appropriate management [6]. One common chameleon that the author observed is vertigo that is commonly mistaken for benign positional vertigo (BPV).

References:

1. Ashish Nanda, MD and Chief Editor: Andrew K Chang, MD. Transient Ischemic Attack. [Online] Dec 30, 2018. https://emedicine.medscape.com/article/1910519-overview#a3.
2. Clinical Differentiation: Cortical vs. Subcortical Strokes. [Online] 2004. http://casemed.case.edu/clerkships/neurology/neurlrngobjectives/neurlrngobj_stroke01new.htm.
3. Ashish Nanda, MD and Chief Editor: Andrew K Chang, MD. Transient Ischemic Attack. [Online] Dec 3, 2018. https://emedicine.medscape.com/article/1910519-overview#a3.
4. Edward C Jauch, MD, MS, FAHA, FACEP and Chief Editor: Helmi L Lutsep, MD. Ischemic Stroke Differential Diagnoses. [Online] Jan 31, 2019. https://emedicine.medscape.com/article/1916852-differential.
5. *Clinical features of stroke mimics in the emergency department.* Yuichi Okano, Kazuaki Ishimatsu, Yoichi Kato. 3: 241-248, s.l. : Acute Med Surg., 2018, Vol. 5.
6. *Clinical Distinction ofCerebral Ischemia andTriaging of Patients in theEmergency DepartmentMimics, Wake-ups, Late Strokes, andChameleons.* Shannon Hextrum, MD José Biller,MD. s.l. : Neuroimag Clin N Am, 2018, Vol. 28.
7. *Stroke chameleons: Uncommon presentations of a common disease.* Pushpendra Nath Renjen, Dinesh Chaudhari. 3, s.l. : Apollo Medcicne, 2017, Vol. 14.

4

Atherosclerosis & Other Cerebrovascular Diseases

▪ Atherosclerosis

Atherosclerosis is a disease of the arterial wall. It is the most common vascular injury that can lead to ischemic strokes. It is a chronic progressive condition in which arteries harden through build-up of plaques. The classic risk factors for atherosclerosis include high cholesterol (hypercholesterolemia), diabetes mellitus (DM), cigarette smoking, hypertension and genetic abnormalities. Stroke results from either mechanical obstruction of flow when atherosclerotic disease causes hemodynamically significant narrowing or from thrombus formation (on the diseased segment) that travels to a more distal arterial bed.

Hypercholesterolemia impairs arterial endothelial integrity by increasing permeability which allows lipids (LDL-C) into the arterial wall (subendothelial space). This change triggers monocytes to adhere to the endothelial cells and, consequently, enter into the subendothelial space and convert into foamy macrophages. LDL particles are oxidized and become strong attractants. These processes only enhance the accumulation of massive intracellular cholesterol by attracting more macrophages which bind native and modified lipoproteins and anionic phospholipids (Table 4.1 and Figure 4.1). Clinical sequelae of atherosclerosis are narrowing and sometimes thrombosis due to plaque instability [1].

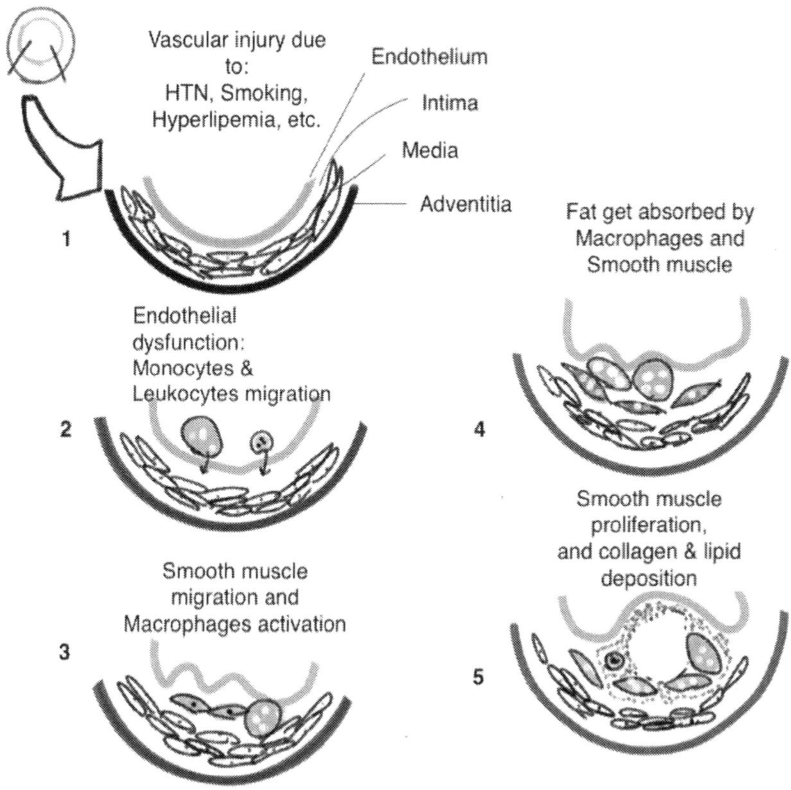

Figure 4.1. The cascade of events leading to atherosclerosis.

From a practical standpoint, cerebrovascular atherosclerosis is divided into cervical atherosclerotic disease (CAD) and intra-cranial atherosclerotic disease (ICAD). CAD is more common in Caucasians, while ICAD is more common in Asians. The natural history of asymptomatic vs. symptomatic

ICAD differs from that of CAD. Compared to asymptomatic extracranial carotid disease, asymptomatic ICAD has a low risk of stroke, while the risk is very high in patients with symptomatic ICAD, especially early after a stroke in patients with clinically significant hemodynamic stenosis [2].

Table 4.1. Atherosclerosis stages.

Vascular modifications in atherosclerotic disease [1]	
Intimal thickening	Layers of smooth muscles and extracellular matrix More frequent in coronary artery, carotid artery, abdominal aorta, descending aorta, and iliac artery
Fatty streak	Abundant macrophage foam cells mixed with smooth muscles and proteoglycan-rich intima
Pathologic intimal thickening	Layers of sooth muscles in proteoglycan-collagen matrix aggregated near the lumen Underlying lipid pool: acellular area rich in hyaluronan and proteoglycans with lipid infiltrates
Fibroatheromas	Acellular necrotic core (cellular debris) Necrotic core is covered by a thick fibrous cap: smooth muscles and proteoglycan-collagen matrix
Vulnerable plaque	'Thin-cap fibroatheroma' Type I collagen, very few/absent sooth muscles Fibrous cap thickness is $\leq 65\,\mu m$
Ruptured plaque	Ruptured fibrous cap Presence of luminal thrombus Larger necrotic core and increased macrophage infiltration of the thin fibrous cap

▪ Arterial dissection

The arterial wall has three different layers (intima, media, adventitia). A tear in the artery inner wall, the intima, can lead to dissection. If deep enough, this dissection can allow blood to leak through the tear and in between the layers of the wall. The deeper the tear, the higher the dissection grade and the lower the chance of spontaneous healing. Table 4.2 and Figure 4.2 show different grades of arterial dissection. As the blood accumulates in the area of the dissection (false lumen), it forms a clot and mass effect on the true inner lumen that reduces blood flow through the narrowed area. If the clot is large enough to completely block blood flow, this can result in an ischemic stroke. It is considered equally dangerous, when pieces of the clot break off and travel up through the bloodstream with resultant blood flow obstruction to the brain and stroke. Like atherosclerosis, arterial dissection is divided into cervical arterial dissection and intracranial arterial dissection.

Cervical artery dissection can involve carotid or vertebral arteries and sometimes multiple arteries at the same time. It is more common than intracranial dissection. There are multiple risk factors for spontaneous dissection such as Marfan, vascular Ehler-Danlos syndromes (connective tissue disease), fibromuscular dysplasia and even atherosclerosis.

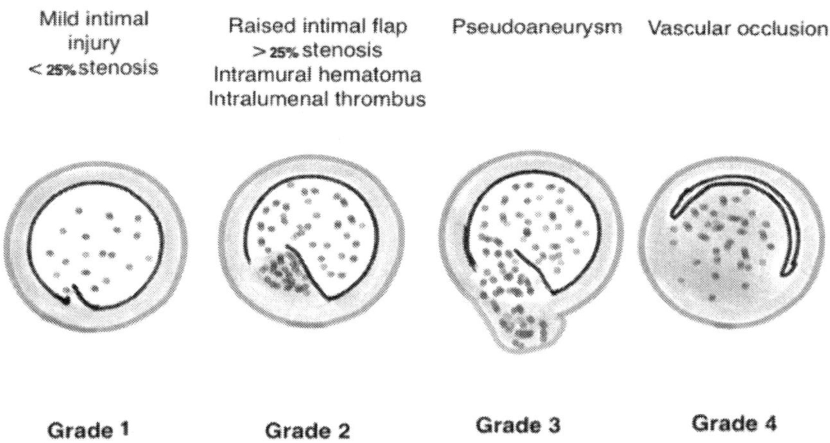

Figure 4.2. Arterial dissection grading system.

Table 4.2. Arterial dissection grading system.

Arterial Dissection Grading System (3)		
	Description	**Treatment and prognosis**
Grade 1	mild intimal injury or irregular intima	heals regardless of therapy
Grade 2	dissection with raised intimal flap / intramural hematoma with luminal narrowing >25% / intraluminal thrombosis	70% of dissections or hematomas with luminal stenosis progress while on therapy
Grade 3	pseduoaneurysm	only ~8% of pseudoaneurysms heal with medical treatment and ~90% resolve after stenting
Grade 4	vessel occlusion/thrombosis	occluded carotid arteries do not recanalize in the early post-injury period
Grade 5	vessel transection	transactions are lethal and refractory to therapy

Traumatic neck and head injury are major risk factors for cervical and intracranial dissection. It can occur due to blunt injury to the neck, such as a high-speed car accident, fall, chiropractic manipulation, or from hyperextension of the neck in sports or exercise. Cervical dissection has also been reported after heavy weight lifting. In addition to the previously listed conditions, high blood pressure and smoking increase the risk of cervical dissection. Also, invasive diagnostic procedures can cause "iatrogenic" dissection.

Dissecting pseudoaneurysms do not always form immediately after initial dissection. They can form at a later stage. They are not benign, especially if they occur intracranially where they carry a very high risk of rupture and subarachnoid hemorrhage. At the cervical level they rarely rupture, but they may compress surrounding structures.

Most common symptoms of dissection are headache, ipsilateral neck and facial pain (mainly around eye), double vision or a droopy eyelid, a pulsatile whooshing "tinnitus" sound in ipsilateral ear or decrease in taste. Though dissection causes local and referred pain (in the neck mainly), sometimes stroke is the first presentation of cervical artery dissection where emergency treatment is required. Symptoms usually develop over hours or days after dissection.

Stroke symptoms can develop hours, days or even a week after these symptoms begin. Anterior circulation strokes that result from carotid artery dissection, and posterior circulation strokes that result from vertebral artery dissection, have the same pattern seen in cortical strokes syndrome discussed in chapter 2.

▪ Vasculopathies

There are many rare cerebral vasculopathies that are associated with stroke. Identification of these disorders has important implications for prevention and treatment as well as allowing identification of other family members at risk. The scope of this book is not to discuss in detail these conditions. Fabry disease, homocystinuria, Menkes disease and the mitochondrial disorders and early atherosclerosis due to genetic hyperlipidemias and Tangier disease are some examples [(4)].

There are many collagen vascular disorders that increase risk of arterial dissection such as Loeys–Dietz syndrome, Marfan syndrome, Ehlers–Danlos syndrome type IV, and pseudoxanthoma elasticum [4].

Moya Moya syndrome is an aggressive cerebrovascular disorder. It has been associated in a variety of inherited disorders such as sickle cell anemia, neurofibromatosis type I, and Down and Williams syndromes. CADASIL and CARASIL are very aggressive small vessel vasculopathies that affect younger patients [4].

More detailed discussion about these vasculopathies is not in the scope of this book.

Cerebral vasculitis

Patients presenting with multi-focal symptoms (due to ischemic or hemorrhagic strokes) along with headache, psychiatric symptoms and signs of a systemic inflammatory disorder need a diagnostic work-up (such as ESR, CRP, CBC) for cerebral vasculitis. Vasculitis can be isolated (primary angitis of CNS; PACNS) or part of a systemic disease. CNS vasculitis should be differentiated from a more benign condition, reversible cerebral vasoconstriction (RCVS) (Table 4.3). The confirmatory standard tests are cerebral angiogram and biopsy [5].

Table 4.3. Differential diagnosis between PACNS and RCVS.

Differential diagnosis between primary angiitis of the central nervous system (PACNS) and reversible cerebral vasoconstriction syndrome (RCVS) [5]		
	RCVS	**PACNS**
Feature	Recurrent thunderclap headache	Insidious, chronic headache
Infarct pattern	Watershed	Small, scattered
Cortical ICH	Common	Very rare
Lobar ICH	Common	Very rare
Reversible edema	Common	Possible
Angiography	Sausage on a string sign	Irregular, notched, ectasia

▪ Cerebral venous thrombosis (CVT)

Thrombosis of the cerebral venous system is an uncommon cause of cerebral infarction and bleed with potential morbidity. It often affects young adults, women of childbearing age, and children. The most common clinical manifestations are headache, seizures, altered consciousness, and neurological focal signs on physical examination. Although the mortality rate of CVT has been significantly reduced by improvements in treatment and diagnostic techniques, the mortality rate of severe CVT remains as high as 34.2%. Survivors of this type of CVT have varying degrees of residual symptoms and are not able to return to their previous work [(6)].

Common locations for cerebral infarction are superior sagittal sinus lateral sinus, and sigmoid sinus. Like ischemic arterial stroke, venous infarction symptoms are related to the area of thrombosis [(6)].

Lateral sinus thrombosis may be associated with headache and a pseudotumor cerebri–like picture. Extension into the jugular bulb may cause jugular foramen syndrome, while cranial nerve palsies may be seen in cavernous sinus thrombosis as a compressive phenomenon. Cerebral hemorrhage also may be a presenting feature in patients with venous sinus thrombosis [(7)].

Common causes of CVT

Many causes have been identified in CVT. These may be seen alone or in combination. Prothrombin gene mutation in association with oral contraceptives are considered risk factors for CVT. Other causes are the following [(7)]:

Sinusitis: Frontal sinuses are the most common source of infection that causes CVT. Multiple organisms are to be considered, with *Staphylococcus aureus* being the most common.

Trauma and surgery: CVT can result from minor head trauma and neurosurgical procedures such as dural taps and injections into the internal jugular vein.

Hypercoagulable states: CVT can occur in antiphospholipid syndrome, protein S and C deficiencies, antithrombin III deficiency, lupus anticoagulant, and the Factor V Leiden mutation. Antibodies against the fibrinolytic receptor, annexin A2 (titer >3 standard deviations), are significantly associated with CVT. Pregnancy and malignancies may be associated with hypercoagulable states that contribute to CVT.

Medications such as oral contraceptives, corticosteroids, epsilon-aminocaproic acid, thalidomide, tamoxifen, erythropoietin, phytoestrogens, L-asparaginase, and heparin (in HIT) may cause CVT.

References

1. *Pathophysiology and treatment of atherosclerosis Current view and future perspective on lipoprotein modification treatment.* S. C. Bergheanu, M. C. Bodde, and J. W. Jukemacorresponding author. 4, s.l. : Neth Heart J, 2017, Vol. 25.
2. *Intracranial Atherosclerosis: Current Understanding and Perspectives.* author, Oh Young Bangcorresponding. 1, s.l. : J Stroke, 2014, Vol. 16.
3. Craig Hacking, MD, Ki Yap, MD. Biffl scale for blunt cerebrovascular injury. [Online] https://radiopaedia.org/articles/biffl-scale-for-blunt-cerebrovascular-injury.
4. *New insights into the pathogenesis of pseudoxanthoma elasticum and related soft tissue calcification disorders by identifying genetic interactions and modifiers.* Hendig D, Knabbe C, Götting C. 114, s.l. : Frontiers in Genetics, 2013, Vol. 4.
5. *Cerebral vasculitis in adults: what are the steps in order to establish the diagnosis? Red flags and pitfalls.* Kraemer, P Berlit and M. s.l. : Clin Exp Immunol, 2014, Vols. 3 (419-424).
6. *Diagnosis and Treatment of Cerebral Venous Thrombosis: A Review.* Yaxi Luo, Xin Tian, Xuefeng Wang. 2, s.l. : Front. Aging Neurosci, 2018, Vol. 10.
7. W Alvin McElveen, MD and Chief Editor: Helmi L Lutsep, MD. Cerebral Venous Thrombosis. [Online] Oct 09, 2018. https://emedicine.medscape.com/article/1162804-overview.

5

Stroke Detection and Triage (Pre-Hospital)

▪ Patients and family

Public education about stroke is at the highest importance nowadays especially since acute stroke is a time-sensitive disease and has a huge burden on healthcare system and economy. The public should be extensively educated about stroke risk factors, signs and symptoms, diagnosis, treatment and prevention.

There are multiple sources that can be used in this regard (https://www.cdc.gov/stroke/docs/ConsumerEd_Stroke.pdf). Stroke centers should utilize all available resources and local health promotion organizations to spread the message. There should be outreach campaigns to increase awareness of stroke symptoms to more rapidly engage EMS and improve time to treatment. The most commonly promoted stroke detection tool for the public is FAST that will be discussed later in this chapter.

▪ EMS triaging tools (stroke scales)

Stroke detection tools

Rapid identification of acute stroke is paramount in order to implement emergent treatment and attain good outcome. EMS

Table 5.1. Cincinnati Prehospital Stroke Scale.

CPSS/FAST	Cincinnati Prehospital Stroke Scale	
F	**Facial droop (Ask the patient to show their teeth or smile)**	
	Normal Both sides of the face move equally	**Abnormal** One side of the face doesn't move as well as the other
A	**Arm drift (Ask the patient to close their eyes and extend both arms straight out for 10 seconds)**	
	Normal Both arms move the same, or both arms don't move at all	**Abnormal** One arm either doesn't move, or one arm drifts down compared to the other
S	**Speech (Ask the patient to repeat the phrase, "The sky is blue in Cincinnati")**	
	Normal The patient says the correct phrase with no slurring of words.	**Abnormal** The patient slurs words say the wrong words or is unable to speak.
T	**Time to call 911**	

personnel are the first line of defense. Local and national organizations should help raise public awareness for stroke symptoms, risk factors, and treatment. These efforts are most successful when they target the general public as well as professionals such as EMS providers.

EMS should be equipped with easy and reliable stroke assessment tool. The National Institute of Health Stroke Scale (NIHSS) is well-recognized as the standard for assessing stroke severity.However, it is time consuming and requires experience and thus it is not practical for use during the pre-hospital assessment by EMS personnel. Current guidelines recommend that EMS utilize validated instruments such as the FAST scale, Los Angeles Prehospital Stroke Screen (LAPSS), Miami Emergency

Table 5.2. Los Angeles Prehospital Stroke Screen

<table>
<tr><th colspan="10">Los Angeles Prehospital Stroke Screen (LAPSS)</th></tr>
<tr><th>Screening Criteria</th><th>Y</th><th>N</th><th>Un-known</th><th>Facial Smile/ Grimace</th><th>Grip</th><th>Arm Strength</th><th></th><th>Y</th><th>N</th></tr>
<tr><td>1.Age over 45 years</td><td></td><td></td><td></td><td rowspan="6">Normal
Droop (R)
Droop (L)</td><td rowspan="6">Normal
Weak grip (R)
Weak grip (L)
No grip (R)
No grip (L)</td><td rowspan="6">Normal
Drifts down (R)
Drifts down (L)
Falls rapidly (R)
Falls rapidly (L)</td><td>Based on exam, patient has only unilateral (and not bilateral) weakness:</td><td></td><td></td></tr>
<tr><td>2.History of seizures or epilepsy absent</td><td></td><td></td><td></td><td>7. If Yes (or unknown) to all items above LAPSS screening criteria met:</td><td></td><td></td></tr>
<tr><td>3.Symptom duration < 24 hours</td><td></td><td></td><td></td><td colspan="3" rowspan="4">If LAPSS criteria for stroke are met, call receiving hospital with "CODE STROKE", if not then return to the appropriate treatment protocol.

(Note: the patient may still be experiencing a stroke even if LAPSS criteria are not met)</td></tr>
<tr><td>4. At baseline, patient is not wheelchair bound or bedridden</td><td></td><td></td><td></td></tr>
<tr><td>5. Blood glucose between 60 and 400</td><td></td><td></td><td>N/A</td></tr>
<tr><td>6. Exam: Look for obvious asymmetry</td><td></td><td></td><td>N/A</td></tr>
</table>

Neurologic Deficit Checklist (MENDC) or Cincinnati Prehospital Stroke Scale (CPSS) (Table 5.1). Most of the prehospital stroke assessment tools can be performed in less than one minute. The CPSS and FAST has a sensitivity of 83% and 85% and a specificity of 69% and 68%, respectively in detecting stroke [(1)].

The American Stroke Association (ASA) promotes the FAST campaign, an acronym constructed to instruct individuals to evaluate for **F**acial droop, **A**rm weakness, and **S**peech difficulty, and if these deficits are found, it's **T**ime to call 9-1-1. Tables 5.1 and 5.2 explain CPSS/FAST and LAPSS.

Severe stroke or LVO

Due to advancement of acute stroke therapy and increasingly available comprehensive stroke centers (CSC) or thrombectomy capable stroke centers (TCSC), there is increased need for more accurate scales that can reliably identify patients with severe strokes due to large vessel occlusion (LVO) who are candidates for endovascular treatment (EVT). Identifying these subset of stroke patients immediately in field and transporting them directly to nearest CSC or TCSC with EVT capabilities saves more neurons and improves outcome [(2) (3)].

The new robust evidence about the benefit of rapid EVT in patients with acute ischemic stroke (AIS) due to LVO has been challenging prehospital systems around the world. Healthcare systems cannot afford to miss suitable candidates anymore. Recent figures show eligibility of ~25% for thrombolysis and ~10% for EVT in all AIS arriving at the hospital within 24 hours [(2) (3)].

Though there are many scales to serve this purpose, current national guidelines have not yet embraced a requirement for use of a prehospital LVO scale (Table 5.3). Fortunately, many state legislations have identified this need in order to filter appropriate patients to CSC or TCSC centers.

Table 5.3. Large vessel occlusion (LVO) scales.

Overview of Several Scores Tested for LVO Prediction in AIS [1]			
Simple Scores (Paramedics)	**Cutoff**	**Complex Scores (Stroke Physicians or Nurses)**	**Cutoff**
The Cincinnati Stroke Triage Assessment Tool (C-STAT)	≥1	RACE	≥2
Los Angeles Motor Scale (LAMS)	≥4	Full NIHSS	≥7
Prehospital Acute Stroke Severity (PASS)	≥2	ASTRAL-occlusion score	≥13
Gaze-Face-Arm-Speech-Time (G-FAST)	≥3		
Vision, Aphasia, Neglect (VAN)	Patient must have weakness plus one or all of the V, A, or N to be VAN positive		positive

The cutoffs to achieve a false-negative rate are ~10% according to current research. At these cutoffs, there is always a significant false-positive rate (overdiagnosis) of LVO. Most scores still need prehospital validation. AIS indicates acute ischemic stroke; ASTRAL, Acute Stroke Registry and Analysis of Lausanne; LVO, large vessel occlusion; NIHSS, National Institute of Health Stroke Scale; and RACE, Rapid Arterial Occlusion Evaluation.

NIHSS cutoff for a low false-negative rate may be lower in certain studies and at later time windows.

Table. 5.4. Rapid Arterial oCclusion Evaluation (RACE)

Rapid Arterial oCclusion Evaluation (RACE) [4]		
Item	**Race Score**	**NIHSS Score Equivalent**
Facial palsy Absent Mild Moderate to severe	 0 1 2	 0 1 2-3
Arm motor function Normal to mild Moderate Severe	 0 1 2	 0-1 2 3-4
Leg motor function Normal to mild Moderate Severe	 0 1 2	 0-1 2 3-4
Head and gaze deviation Absent Present	 0 1	 0 1-2
Aphasia (if right hemiparesis) Performs both tasks correctly Performs 1 task correctly Performs neither tasks correctly	 0 1 2	 0 1 2
Agnosia Patient recognizes his/her arm and the impairment Does not recognized his/her arm or the impairment Does not recognize his/her arm nor the impairment	 0 1 2	 0 1 2
Score total	0-9	

FAL: face, arm, leg. V: vision. N: neglect. T: talking ability. U: understanding ability. G: gaze

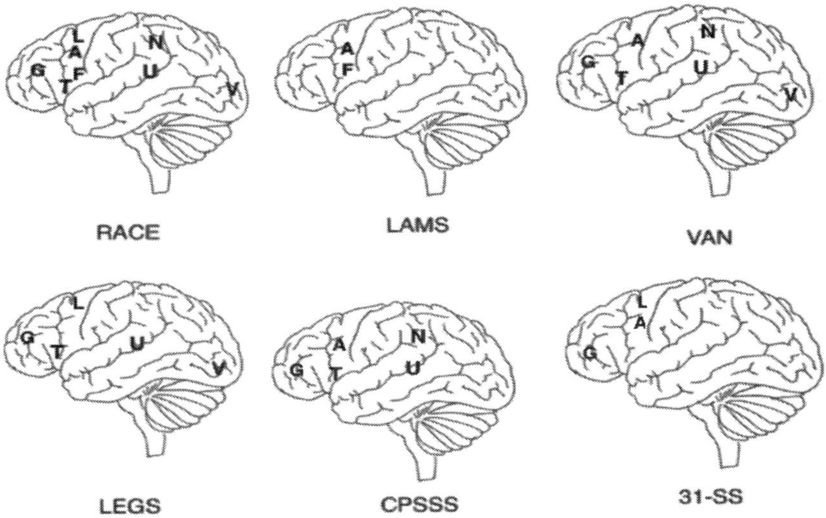

Figure 5.1. Many different large vessel occlusion (LVO) scales. RACE and VAN are the most comprehensive scales.

Among the many LVO scales available (Figure 5.1), RACE (Table 5.4) is the most promising one and potentially has the highest correlation with NIHSS. Another promising scale is VAN scale and it is still under validation process.

ABCs of acute stroke

Once it has been determined that the patient has stroke-like symptoms and after stabilizing basic life functions (ABCs), it is important to obtain a brief history, perform basic necessary examination, and begin transport to a facility capable of definitive therapy.

EMS personnel should ensure "ABCs" of basic life support, (Airway, Breathing, and Circulation). There are additional ABCs that need to be addressed before transportation.

Airway (A)

It is not uncommon that stroke victims have decreased level of consciousness, vomiting with risk of aspiration, agitation and confusion with safety concerns. These conditions might require intubation and sedation. Along with securing airways, EMS personnel should secure IV access (preferably two 18-gauge IVs proximal to the wrist) in order to support IV contrast power infusion. It is also helpful to start intravenous normal saline at a rate of 75 ml/hour if there are no signs of fluid retention.

Blood pressure (BP)

BP value plays a significant role in outcome in ischemic stroke. High BP affects patient outcome and may delay IV alteplase (tPA) administration. The author strongly recommends that prior to hospital arrival all suspected stroke patients have a systolic BP 90-180 mmHg (preferably 140-160 mmHg). This is controversial. However, the author recommends this range to cover the possibility of ICH or SAH where lower BP value is preferred. This also saves time needed to control BP in patients who are candidates for IV tPA. EMS can use IV nicardipine (3 mg/hour and titrate) or IV labetalol to achieve this goal.

Blood glucose concentration (C)

Point-of-care testing for glucose can help rule out hypoglycemia as a common stroke mimic. Low blood sugar and high blood sugar in patients with suspected acute stroke should be addressed and treated immediately. High blood sugar treatment can wait until arrival to hospital if EMS personnel are not equipped and / or not trained with insulin.

History

While or after addressing the ABCs, EMS personnel should obtain a focused history without delaying transportation. Particular attention should be paid to the last time the patient is known to be well (last known well, LKW). It is very helpful to bring a family member in the ambulance to the ED. This helps avoid delay in confirmation of LKW time and allows prompt initiation of reperfusion therapy. A patient who woke up with new symptoms (wake up stroke), LKW should be considered at the last time he or she was last seen awake. Additionally, a medication list, with focus on anti-coagulation, should be obtained.

Despite evidence about the harmful effect of persistent hyperglycemia (>140 mg / dL) during the first 24 hours, EMS personnel should focus on treating hypoglycemia. If EMS is not well equipped to deal with hyperglycemia, treatment may be deferred to the emergency room doctor.

One of the most important components of stroke care that EMS can provide is a pre-notification report to the receiving hospital. Pre-notification allows the receiving institution to activate local protocols, prepare necessary medications, prepare and hold the CT scanner, and be prepared to assess the patient immediately upon arrival [(5) (6)].

▪ Communication tools (SSS)

It has been proven that EMS hospital pre-notification improves evaluation, time of stroke treatment, and increases the number of eligible patients who receives thrombolytics.

The author has worked with multiple hospital systems in different geographic areas and based on extensive evidence, proposes the SSS system: **S**imultaneous communication, **S**tandardized communication, and **S**how / share results.

Simultaneous communication

When communication happens in sequence (EMS to ED charge nurse, charge nurse to stroke nurse or physician, ED to stroke / interventional physician) information is likely to get lost and critical time-sensitive information does not get conveyed to the treating team, especially neurointerventional team, in timely fashion. Since it is impossible to have simultaneous conversation with multiple team members at the same time, it is very useful to use electronic communication methods to ensure simultaneous informed communication.

There are many EMS mobile communication applications that can be used to achieve this goal. These applications can also transmit videos and images that help treating physicians with getting more accurate clinical picture. This may help in early activation of the neuorinterventional team. These communication applications can also be used to provide estimate time of arrival and any changes in patient condition. Ideally, they should allow 2-way communication, so treating physicians can ask questions and provide further recommendations and instructions to EMS personnel.

Standardized communication

Every stroke team should establish effective communication with EMS leaders in the geographic area they serve. Discussion should focus on what information is most useful to collect and convey to the treating team and what initial measures are needed to stabilize patients prior to ED arrival. Standardizing reports and handoffs improve communication, reduce mistakes, and minimize false positive and false negative stroke alerts.

This report ideally should include the following (**ABCCD PARTSS**):

1. **A**irway status
2. **B**lood pressure
3. **C**onsciousness level (if not included in stroke scale)
4. **C**ontact information of family or guardian
5. **D**rugs especially anticoagulants
6. **P**ast medical history
7. **A**ge
8. **R**ecording for borderline cases (live streaming video)
9. **T**ime of last known well (LKW)
10. **S**ex
11. **S**troke scale used and score

Show/Share results

In the author's experience, it is frustrating to EMS personnel and ED team that they rarely find out what happens to a patient after stroke team takes over care. Showing or sharing results with EMS and other team members has a very positive impact on the process and on team building. Closing the loop helps make everyone involved in stroke care feel like they are part of a team within a system of care, encouraging further collaboration and cooperation [5]. Providing near real-time feedback is the best way to continuously improve and gain the confidence needed to make those lifesaving decisions again and again for these patients [5].

Stroke center designations

Determining destination hospital

It is of highest importance to field stroke patients to be transported to the most appropriate hospital capable of providing the highest level of stroke care. Regional stroke stakeholders should develop regional fielding / triaging plan for EMS personnel to follow in order to streamline the process and create very efficient and easily reproducible triaging process [6].

There are four levels of stroke center designations: acute stroke ready hospitals (ASRH), primary stroke center (PSC), thrombectomy ready center (TRC), and comprehensive stroke center (CSC). It is very important for EMS to understand the differences amongst these four designations [7].

Acute stroke ready hospitals (ASRH) are hospitals that have the following components:

1. The ability to perform diagnostic imaging and laboratory tests 24/7 with results within 45 minutes.
2. Access to stroke expertise 24/7 (in person or via telemedicine) and transfer protocols with facilities that provide primary or comprehensive stroke services.
3. The ability to administer intravenous thrombolytics, if needed, prior to transferring the patient to a facility that provides primary or comprehensive stroke services.

Primary stroke centers (PSC) are hospitals that have the following components:

1. Dedicated stroke-focused program and staffing by qualified medical professionals trained in stroke care.
2. Individualized care to meet stroke patients' needs.
3. Patient involvement in their hospital care.
4. Coordination of post-discharge patient self-care based on recommendations of the Brain Attack Coalition and guidelines published by the American Heart Association/American Stroke Association or equivalent guidelines.
5. Streamlined flow of patient information while protecting patients' rights, security, and privacy.
6. Collection of the hospital's stroke-treatment performance data.
7. Hospital team performance data.
8. Use of data to assess and continually improve quality of care for stroke patients.

Thrombectomy capable stroke centers (TCSC) are hospitals that have the following components:

1. Must have performed mechanical thrombectomy and post-procedure care for at least 15 patients with ischemic stroke in the past 12 months or at least 30 patients over the past 24 months.
2. Demonstrate compliance with the new standards for TCSC certification.
3. Meet the minimum mechanical thrombectomy volume requirement.
4. Demonstrate the ability to perform mechanical thrombectomy 24/7.
5. Maintain dedicated intensive care beds for acute ischemic stroke patients.
6. Meet the expectations for the availability of staff and practitioners closely aligned with CSC expectations.

7. Collect and review data regarding adverse patient outcomes following mechanical thrombectomy.
8. Collect data for 13 standardized performance measures.

Comprehensive stroke centers (CSC) are hospitals that have all components of PSC in addition to the following:

1. Availability of advanced imaging techniques, including MRI/MRA, CTA, DSA and TCD.
2. Availability of personnel trained in vascular neurology, neurosurgery and endovascular procedures.
3. 24/7 availability of personnel, imaging, operating room and endovascular facilities.
4. ICU/neuroscience ICU facilities and capabilities.
5. Experience and expertise treating patients with large ischemic strokes, intracerebral hemorrhage and subarachnoid hemorrhage.

As the highest level of stroke center designation, CSCs are the most capable centers of taking care of not only ischemic stroke patients, but also hemorrhagic stroke and subarachnoid hemorrhage (SAH) patients.

The decision where to take acute ischemic stroke patients after being assessed by EMS personnel is very often not straight forward. All hospitals and EMS systems in a certain geographic region should come together and create triaging protocols for all EMS services to follow.

These protocols should be based on the fact that "time is brain". The protocol should include standardized triaging tool/scale and preferred center based on stroke severity (LVO or no LVO), time of LKW, distance from field to stroke centers, and distance between stroke centers with different levels of designation. The team should keep in mind that CSCs are more efficient in delivering IV tPA and obtaining advanced imaging than all other centers including PSCs. Our EMS' recommended field triage protocol is summarized in table 5.5 and will be discussed again in chapter 7.

Table 5.5. Recommended triaging protocol based on stroke severity, time from LKW, and level of designation of receiving hospital.

Proposed triaging based on level of designation				
	Mild stroke		**Sever stroke**	
Hospital designation	**NIHSS < 4 No LVO 0-4.5 hours from LKW**	**NIHSS < 4 No LVO 4.5-24 hours from LKW**	**NIHSS > 4 Yes LVO 0-4.5 hours from LKW**	**NIHSS > 4 Yes LVO 4.5-24 hours from LKW**
ASRH	-Triage to nearest ASRH if PSC or CSC is > 45 minutes away -Transfer to nearest PSC or CSC (whichever is closer) after tPA			
PSCs	-Triage directly to PSC (or CSC whichever is closer) if PSC or CSC is < 45 minutes away	-Triage to nearest PSC or CSC (whichever is closer)	-Triage to nearest PSC first if CSC is > 45 minutes to receive IV tPA -Transfer to CSC after starting tPA (drip & ship)	
CSC/ TCSC		-Triage to nearest CSC/TCSC if not sure stroke is mild	-Triage to nearest CSC/TCSC if within 45 minutes distance	-Triage to nearest CSC/TCSC
All suspected bleed especially SAH should be transferred directly to CSC.				

References

1. *Prehospital Scales for Large Vessel Occlusion: Closing in on a Moving Target.* Michel, Patrik. s.l. : Stroke, 2017, Vols. 48 (247-249).
2. *Organizational Update: European Stroke Organisation.* Caso V, Fischer U, van der Worp HB. 3, s.l. : Stroke, 2015, Vol. 46.
3. *Comparison of stroke recognition and stroke severity scores for stroke detection in a single cohort.* Purrucker JC, Hametner C, Engelbrecht A. 9, s.l. : J Neurol Neurosurg Psychiatry., 2015, Vol. 86.
4. *Design and Validation of a Prehospital Stroke Scale to Predict Large Arterial OcclusionThe Rapid Arterial Occlusion Evaluation Scale.* Natalia Pérez de la Ossa, MD, PhD and David Carrera, MD. s.l. : Stroke, 2014, Vol. 45.
5. James Woodson, MD , E. Stein Bronsky, MD. Effective Communication In EMS. [Online] Jan 2, 2018. https://www.jems.com/articles/print/volume-43/issue-1/features/effective-communication-in-ems.html.
6. Henry G. Colmer IV, MD , Elizabeth K. Powell, MD , Natalie Kreitzer, MD. *Acute Stroke: From Prehospital Care to In-Hospital Management.* [Online] , May 1, 2018. https://www.jems.com/articles/print/volume-43/issue-5/features/acute-stroke-from-prehospital-care-to-in-hospital-management.html.
7. Facts about Joint Commission stroke certification. [Online] Sep 2108. https://www.jointcommission.org/facts_about_joint_commission_stroke_certification/.

6

Stroke Detection and Triage (ED)

Stroke triaging protocols

Early recognition of stroke by clinical presentation and prehospital stroke assessment tools facilitates rapid prehospital and ED diagnosis and triage. Appropriate recognition and speedy work up are essential to improve stroke patient outcomes. This also allows safe and prompt administration of advanced specialized treatment, in the hopes of further reducing morbidity and mortality in stroke patients.

After EMS providers determine the most appropriate hospital for a particular stroke patient according to the protocol discussed in Table 5.5, notification (including ABCCD PARTSS discussed in chapter 5) should be sent immediately to the hospital treating teams who in turn should get prepared to meet the patient and EMS providers upon arrival in the ED.

The patient should pass through ED to a pre-determined CT scan suite. ED team should meet the patient immediately and travel with him/her to CT suite and obtain all the information from EMS provider without stopping or delaying the scan. ED providers should reexamine the patient quickly and communicate any significant changes to stroke/interventional team. Also, ED providers should verify all the key elements of the history that EMS conveyed to the teams.

The National Institutes of Health (NIH) provides clear guidelines for initial assessment and interventions. The patient should be evaluated by the ED provider within 10 minutes. Initial NIHSS score should be obtained prior to administering IV tPA. Obtaining NIHSS should not delay IV tPA administration. NIHSS is an essential part that should be obtained accurately and communicated effectively to stroke/neurointerventional team to enable them to weigh benefits and risks more accurately before deciding on IV tPA or endovascular treatment (EVT). The stroke consultant (team) should be notified within 15 minutes. ED physician along with stroke team should determine candidacy for IV tPA.

The patient should have brain non-contrast CT (NCCT) scan initiated by 25 minutes. NCCT and laboratory results should be interpreted within 45 minutes, and IV tPA should be administered if the patient is eligible within 60 minutes (door to needle 60 minutes) of arrival. This is commonly referred to as the "golden hour."

The actual timelines might be variable among hospitals based on level of designation and available resources. Ideally and for best outcome, timelines should be adjusted in order to achieve door to needle time of less than 45 minutes.

NCCT imaging usually consists of a non-contrasted image to evaluate for hemorrhage or other abnormalities. For severe stroke, patient should be kept in CT suite to obtain advanced images if already in CSC or TCSC. However, if patient needs transfer to CSC or TCSC afterward, advanced images is preferably done at the accepting facility where obtaining advanced images is more streamlined and readily available, and reading is prompt. This way, the neurointerventional physician can make decisions based on freshly obtained images, not based on images that were done hours prior to arrival to treating facility.

Advanced imaging consists of CT angiography (CTA) of brain and neck to detect any large vessel occlusion (LVO) that necessitates EVT. However, if the patient presents between 6 and 24 hours, advanced imaging should also include brain CT perfusion to assess penumbra. For most mild strokes (with no LVO signs), there is no need to pursue advanced images such CT angiogram or CT perfusion (CTP) emergently and the focus should be on delivering IV tPA as soon as possible.

While the patient is being triaged and scanned, the team should ensure functional IV access and obtain blood work (if EMS has not done so already). Basic laboratory tests include blood count, basic metabolic panel (mainly creatinine), coagulation function (PT, INR, PTT), and blood glucose. The use of point of care testing (POCT) can save significant amount of time. POCT can check blood glucose, electrolytes (including creatinine), and coagulation (PT/INR).

▪ National Institute of Health Stroke Scale (NIHSS)

NIHSS is made up of 11 different components that assess specific functions (Table 6.1). The score is calculated by adding the number for each component with 42 being the highest score possible. The higher the score, the more severe the stroke. Roughly, a score > 16 predicts higher probability of patient death, while a score of ≤ 6 predicts higher possibility for a good recovery. Each point increase on the scale lowers the possibility of a positive outcome for the patient by 17 %.

▪ Intravenous tissue plasminogen activator (IV tPA)

Patients with an acute ischemic stroke may be eligible for IV tPA within 4.5 hours from time of onset or LKW. IV tPA should not be given beyond 3 hours if: age > 80, history of prior stroke and diabetes, any anticoagulant use prior to admission (even if INR <1.7), NIHSS >25, CT findings involving more than 1/3 of the MCA territory (as evidenced by hypodensity, sulcal effacement or mass effect estimated by visual inspection or ABC/2>100 cc) [(1)].

The decision to administer thrombolytics requires consideration of both inclusion and exclusion criteria discussed in Table 6.2 and chapter 10.

Selecting the right patient with the greatest likelihood of benefit and the least likelihood of harm is important. When deciding on giving IV tPA, the physician should keep in mind and discuss with patient/family that IV tPA carries a 2–6% risk of symptomatic intracranial hemorrhage (sICH). There is no need for written consent as IV tPA is standard of care. Patients who receive tPA may have significant improvement in their stroke symptoms and prevention from permanent disability.

The American College of Emergency Physicians position statement on tPA highlights the importance of regularly balancing the benefits and risks for an individual patient with appropriate patient and family input.

The exclusion criteria for IV tPA are significant head trauma or prior stroke in the last three months, recent surgery, prior intracranial bleeding, very low platelet count, severe hypertension, current use of anticoagulant medications, or known brain cancer (Table 6.2). Additionally, caution is given to patients with very large or devastating strokes, as they are more likely to have a poor outcome [1].

Endovascular treatment (EVT)

For a patient to be a candidate for EVT, there are five criteria that have to be met:

1. Patient is with significant neurological deficit (as judged by interventionist).
2. LKW is within 24 hours.
3. LVO is demonstrated on advanced imaging (CTA) or dense vessel sign on NCCT.
4. Significant mismatch on CTP if > 6 hours from LKW.
5. No evidence of bleed on head CT.

Endovascular therapies involve using a catheter that is threaded from an artery in the groin up to the affected arteries in the brain. The catheter can then be used to manually remove the clot (by stent retriever or aspiration devices) or directly apply tPA to the clot.

Typically, it is preferred that EVT be performed within 6 hours; however, recent publications indicate that the benefit of endovascular therapy may be extended up to 24 hours in patients with favorable CT perfusion findings.

CT perfusion imaging is used to compare the infarct core (the part of the brain that is irreversibly damaged due to the stroke) from the penumbra (the part of the brain that is salvageable). Imaging will be discussed in more detail in chapter 9.

Due to increasing evidence supporting EVT (see chapter 8), all members of treatment team should have basic knowledge about EVT including, time window for treatment, indications and risks, and basic understanding of penumbra. They should be vigilant about LVO signs and confirmatory imaging modalities. It is important to note that eligible patients still receive IV tPA even if EVT is being considered. This will not preclude them from being able to undergo EVT.

The risks associated with EVT mainly include vessel dissection, ischemic stroke, reperfusion hemorrhage and access site complications. More details about EVT complications are discussed in chapter 12. Although it is not considered a risk-free procedure, recent studies have not shown EVT to increase risks above those associated with IV tPA.

Table 6.1. National Institute of Health Stroke Scale (NIHSS)

National Institute of Health Stroke Scale (NIHSS)

Item	Description	Score
1a *Level of consciousness (LOC)*	The investigator must choose a response, even if a full evaluation is prevented by such obstacles as an endotracheal tube, language barrier, orotracheal trauma/bandages. A "3" is scored only if the patient makes no movement (other than reflexive posturing) in response to noxious stimulation.	0 = Alert; keenly responsive 1 = Not alert, but arousable by minor stimulation to obey, answer, or respond 2 = Not alert, requires repeated stimulation to attend, or is obtunded and requires strong or painful stimulation to movements (not stereotyped) 3= Respond only with reflex motor or autonomic effects or totally unresponsive, flaccid, areflexic
1b *LOC questions*	The patient is asked the month and his/her age. The answer must be correct - there is no part credit for being close. Aphasic and stuporous patients who do not comprehend the questions will score "2." Patients unable to speak because of endotracheal intubation, orotracheal trauma, severe dysarthria from any cause, language barrier or any other problem not secondary to aphasia are given a "1." **It is important that only the initial answer be graded and that the examiner not "help" the patient with verbal or non-verbal cues.**	0 = Answers both questions correctly 1 = Answers one question correctly 2 = Answers neither question correctly

2 *Best gaze*	Only horizontal eye movements will be tested. Voluntary or reflexive (oculocephalic) eye movements will be scored but calorie testing is not done. If the patient has a conjugate deviation of the eyes that can be overcome by voluntary or reflexive activity, the score will be "1." If a patient has an isolated peripheral nerve paresis (CN, III, IV or VI) score a "1." Gaze is testable in all aphasic patient. Patients with ocular trauma, bandages, pre-existing blindness or other disorder of visual acuity or fields should be tested with reflexive movements and a choice made by the investigator. Establishing eyes contact and then moving about the patient from side to side will occasionally clarify the presence of a partial gaze palsy.	0= Normal 1= Partial gaze palsy. This score is given when gaze is abnormal in one or both eyes, but where forced deviation or total gaze paresis are not present 2= Forced deviation, or total gaze paresis not overcome by the oculocephalic maneuver

3 *Visual*	Visual fields (upper and lower quadrants) are tested by confrontation, using finger counting or visual threat as appropriate. Patient must be encouraged, but if they look at the side of the moving fingers appropriately, this can be scored as normal. If there is unilateral blindness or enucleation, visual fields in the remaining eye are scored. Score 1 only if a clear-cut asymmetry, including quadrant anopia is found. If patient is blind from any cause, score "3." Double simultaneous stimulation is performed at this point. **If there is extinction, patient receives a "1" and the results are used to answer question #11.**	0 = No visual loss 1= Partial hemianopia 2 = Complete hemianopia 3 = Bilateral hemianopia (blind, including cortical blindness)

4 *Facial palsy*	Ask, or use pantomime to encourage the patient to show teeth or raise eyebrows and close eyes. Score symmetry of grimace in response to noxious stimuli in the poorly responsive or non-comprehending patient. If facial trauma/bandages, orotracheal tube, tape or other physical barrier obscures the face, these should be removed to the extent possible	0 = Normal symmetrical movement 1 = Minor paralysis (flattened nasolabial fold, asymmetry on smiling) 2 = Partial paralysis (total or near total paralysis of lower face) 3 = Complete paralysis of one or both sides (absence of facial movement in the upper and lower face)
5 & 6 *Motor Arm & Leg*	The limb is placed in the appropriate position: extend the arms (palms down) 90 degrees (if sitting) or 45 degrees (if supine) and the leg 30 degrees (always tested supine). Drift is scored if the arm falls before 10 seconds or the leg before 5 seconds. The aphasic patient is encouraged using urgency in the voice and pantomime but not noxious stimulate on. Each limb is tested in turn, beginning with the non-paretic arm. Only in the case of amputation or joint fusion at the shoulder or hip may the score be "9" and the examiner must clearly write the explanation for scoring as a "9"	0 = No drift, limb holds 90 (or 45) degrees for full 10 seconds 1 = Drift, Limb holds 90 (or 45) degrees, but drifts down before full 10 seconds; does not hit bed or other support 2 = Some effort against gravity, limb cannot get to or maintain (if cued) 90 (or 45) degrees, drifts down to bed, but has some effort against gravity 3 = No effort against gravity, limb falls 4 = No movement 9 = Amputation, joint fusion explain: 5a. Left Arm.. 5b. Right Arm..

7 *Limb ataxia*	This item is aimed at finding evidence of a unilateral cerebellar lesion. Test with eyes open. In case of visual defect, insure testing is done in intact visual field. The finger-nose-finger and heel-shin tests are performed on both sides, and ataxia is scored only if present out of proportion to weakness. Ataxia is absent in the patient who cannot understand or is paralyzed. Only in the case of amputation or joint fusion may the item be scored "9", and the examiner must clearly write the explanation for not scoring. In case of blindness test by touching nose from extended arm position	0 = Absent 1 = Present in one limb 2 = Present in two limbs

8 *Sensory*	Sensation or grimace to pin prick when tested, or withdrawal from noxious stimulus in the obtunded or aphasic patient. Only sensory loss attributed to stroke is scored as abnormal and the examiner should test as many body areas [arms (not hands), legs, trunk, face] as needed to accurately check for hemisensory loss. A score of 2, "severe or total," should only be given when a severe or total loss of sensation can be clearly demonstrated. Stuporous and aphasic patients will therefore probably score 1 or 0. The patient with brain stem stroke who has bilateral loss of sensation is scored 2. If the patient does not respond and is quadriplegic score 2. Patients in coma (item 1a=3) are arbitrarily given a 2 on this item	0 = Normal; no sensory loss 1 = Mild to moderate sensory loss; patient feels pinprick is less sharp or is dull on the affected side; or there is a loss of superficial pain with pinprick, but patient is aware he/she is being touched 2 = Severe to total sensory loss; patient is not aware of being touched in the face, arm and leg

9 *Best language*	A great deal of information about comprehension will be obtained during the preceding sections of the examination. The patient is asked to describe what is happening in the attached picture, name the items, and read the sentences. Comprehension is judged from responses here as well as to all of the commands in the preceding general neurological exam. If visual loss interferes with the tests, ask the patient to identify objects placed in the hand, repeat, and produce speech. The intubated patient should be asked to write. The patient in coma (question 1a=3) will arbitrarily score 3 on this item. The examiner must choose a score in the patient with stupor or limited cooperation but a score of 3 should be used only if the patient is mute and follows no one step commands.	0 = No aphasia, normal 1 = Mild to moderate aphasia; some obvious loss of fluency or facility of comprehension, without significant limitation on ideas expressed or form of expression. Reduction of speech and/or comprehension, however, makes conversation about provided material difficult or impossible. For example, in conversation about provided materials examiner can identify picture or naming card from patient's response. 2 = Severe aphasia; all communication is through fragmentary expression; great need for inference, questioning and guessing by the listener. Range of information that can be exchanged is limited; listener carries burden of communication. Examiner cannot identify materials provided from patient response. 3 = Mute, global aphasia; no usable speech or auditory comprehension

10 *Dysarthria*	If patient is thought to be normal an adequate sample of speech must be obtained by asking patient to read or repeat words from the attached list. If the patient has severe aphasia, the clarity of articulation of spontaneous speech can be rated. Only if the patient is intubated or has other physical barrier to producing speech, may the item be scored "9", and the examiner must clearly write an explanation for not scoring. Do not tell the patient why he/she is being tested.	0 = Normal 1 = Mild to moderate; patient slurs at least some words and, at worst, can be understood with some difficulty 2 = Severe; patient's speech is so slurred as to be unintelligible in the absence of or out of proportion to any dysphasia, or is mute/anarthric 9 = Intubated or other physical barrier, explain

11 *Extinction and Inattention*	Sufficient information to identify neglect may be obtained during the prior testing. If the patient has a severe visual loss preventing visual double simultaneous stimulation, and the cutaneous stimuli are normal, the score is normal. If the patient has aphasia but does appear to attend to both sides, the score is normal. The presence of visual spatial neglector anosagnosia may also be taken as evidence of abnormality. Since the abnormality is scored only if present, the item is never untestable	0 = No abnormality 1 = Visual, tactile, auditory, spatial, or personal inattention or extinction to bilateral simultaneous stimulation in one of the sensory modalities 2 = Profound hemi-inattention or hemi-inattention to more than one modality. Does not recognize own hand or orients to only one side of space.

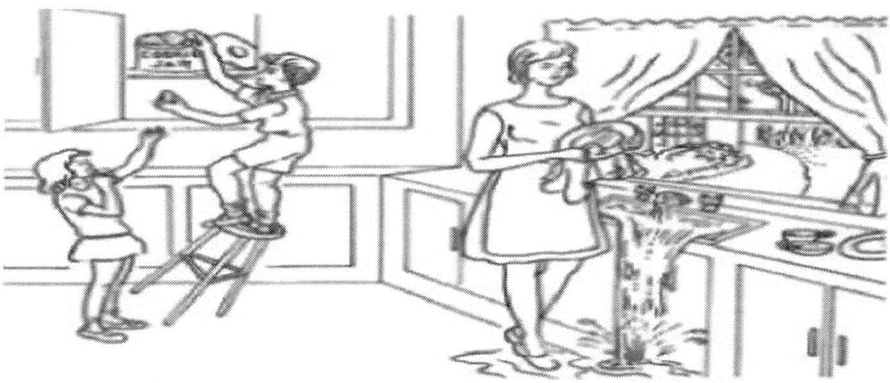

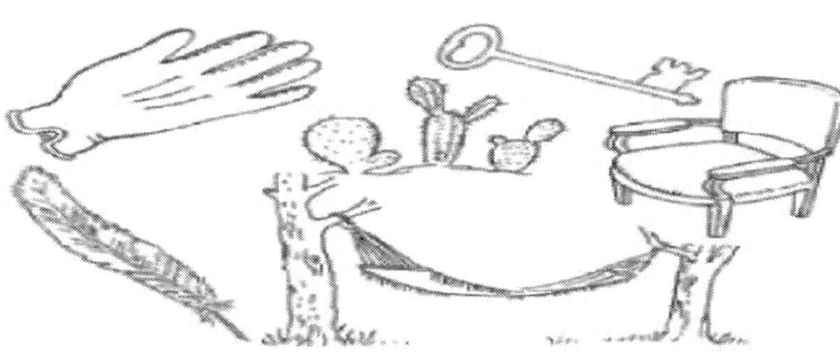

You know how.

Down to earth.

I got home from work.

Near the table in the dining room.

They heard him speak on the radio last night.

MAMA

TIP – TOP

FIFTY – FIFTY

THANKS

HUCKLEBERRY

BASEBALL PLAYER

Table 6.2. Protocol for use of IV tPA within 4.5 hours window.

Inclusion and exclusion criteria for administering IV tPA in acute ischemic stroke (AIS) within 4.5 hours from symptom onset (2)(3)
Inclusion criteria Diagnosis of ischemic stroke causing measurable neurological deficit Onset of symptoms <3 hours before treatment begins Age ≥18 y

Exclusion criteria
Significant head trauma or prior stroke in the previous 3 months
Symptoms suggest SAH
Arterial puncture at non-compressible site in previous 7 days
History of previous intracranial hemorrhage
Intracranial neoplasm, AVM, or aneurysm
Recent intracranial or intraspinal surgery
Elevated blood pressure (systolic >185 mm Hg or diastolic >110 mm Hg)
Active internal bleeding
Acute bleeding diathesis, including but not limited to
    Platelet count <100 000/mm^3
    Heparin received within 48 h resulting in abnormally elevated aPTT above the upper limit of normal
    Current use of anticoagulant with INR >1.7 or PT >15 seconds
    Current use of direct thrombin inhibitors or direct factor Xa inhibitors with elevate sensitive laboratory tests (eg, aPTT, INR, platelet count, ECT, TT, or appropriate factor Xa activity assays)
Blood glucose concentration <50 mg/dL (2.7 mmol/L)
CT demonstrates multilobar infarction (hypodensity >1/3 cerebral hemisphere)
 	
Relative exclusion criteria
Recent experience suggests that under some circumstances, with careful consideration and weighting of risk to benefit, patients may receive fibrinolytic therapy despite ≥1 relative contraindication. Consider risk to benefit of IV tPA administration carefully if any of these relative contraindications is present

- Only minor or rapidly improving stroke symptoms (clearing spontaneously)
- Pregnancy
- Seizure at onset with postictal residual neurological impairments
- Major surgery or serious trauma within previous 14 days
- Recent gastrointestinal or urinary tract hemorrhage (within previous 21 days)
- Recent acute myocardial infarction (within previous 3 months)

Notes

The checklist includes some FDA-approved indications and contraindications for administration of IV tPA for acute ischemic stroke. Recent guideline revisions have modified the original FDA-approved indications. A physician with expertise in acute stroke care may modify this list.

Onset time is defined as either the witnessed onset of symptoms or the time last known normal if symptom onset was not witnessed.

In patients without recent use of OACs or heparin, treatment with IV tPA can be initiated before availability of coagulation test results but should be discontinued if INR is >1.7 or PT is abnormally elevated by local laboratory standards.

In patients without a history of thrombocytopenia, treatment with IV tPA can be initiated before availability of platelet count but should be discontinued if platelet count is <100 000/mm^3

Additional exclusion criteria for 3-4.5 hours window

- Age > 80
- History of prior stroke AND diabetes
- Any anticoagulant use prior to admission (even if INR <1.7)
- NIHSS >25
-]CT findings involving more than 1/3 of the MCA territory (as evidenced by hypodensity, sulcal effacement or mass effect estimated by visual inspection or ABC/2>100 cc)

References:

1. *Randomised double-blind placebo-controlled trial of thrombolytic therapy with intravenous alteplase in acute ischaemic stroke (ECASS II).* . Hacke W, Kaste M, Fieschi C, von Kummer R. 9136, s.l. : Lnacet, 1998, Vol. 352.
2. *Expansion of the Time Window for Treatment of Acute Ischemic Stroke WithIntravenous Tissue Plasminogen Activator. A Science Advisory From the American Heart Association/American StrokeAssociation.* del Zoppo G, Saver J, Jauch EC,. 2945, s.l. : Stroke, 2009, Vol. 40.
3. *Scientific Rationale for the Inclusion and Exclusion Criteria for Intravenous Alteplase in Acute Ischemic A Stroke Statement for Healthcare Professionals From the American Heart Association/American Stroke Association.* Bart M. Demaerschalk, MD, MSc, FRCPC, FAHA, Chair, Dawn O. Kleindorfer, MD, FAHA, Vice-Chair and Opeolu M. Adeoye, MD, MS, FAHA. s.l. : Stroke, 2015, Vol. 47.

7

Stroke Detection and Triage (Stroke Teams and Protocols)

▪ Stroke teams

Acute stroke is one of the most urgent medical emergencies due to a very short treatment window of opportunity. This requires rapid detection, triaging and evaluation in order to implement emergent treatment in timely fashion that leads to good outcome. Establishing stroke teams is critical because it requires a "village" to achieve this purpose. It takes tremendous amount of effort and planning to put an effective stroke team in place. The higher the stroke designation a hospital has, the more sophisticated, collaborative and efficient the stroke team. Good leadership is also key to success.

The structure and number of stroke team members vary depending on the needs of the individual hospital and level of designation. Figure 7.1 shows the different disciplines involved in stroke care. The central area represents stroke core team. Stroke core team is responsible for setting up strategies, protocols and action plans for the rest of the team members. It is very critical that senior-level administration and leadership is on board with stroke core team in order to ensure all needed infrastructures and investments are guaranteed in order to build a functional and complete stroke team.

To achieve maximal efficiency and best outcome possible, all services involved in the care of stroke patients, including the local community, EMS, ED, neurointerventional (NI) services, neurosurgery, nursing, quality department, radiology services, laboratory, pharmacy, rehabilitation, and inpatient units including neuro intensive care unit (NICU) and stroke unit, should be functionally integrated (Figure 7.1). It is very essential to ensure early input and continuous involvement from the hospital's administration during not only establishing the team, but also while program is evolving as operational challenges may unfold after the program becomes busy. Therefore, involvement of senior administration is essential to enhance problem solving and integration between services.

The team should educate the public and care providers about stroke warning signs and about the availability of stroke treatments, evaluate and streamline services, provide stroke treatment rapidly, and continually monitor the efficacy of its work. There should be periodic quality and operational meetings that includes all disciplines' leaders.

Operationally, the team is made up of 2 parts: (1) the stroke code team, who respond to stroke codes and deliver urgent treatment, and (2) stroke support team who take over care after stroke code team deliver urgent treatment. **Stroke code team** consists of a neurologist (or stroke physician), ED physician, ED nurse, CT tech, lab tech, pharmacist, and ECG tech. In CSC, the team may include NICU nurse and NIR physician. **Stroke support team** include members from many disciplines, including rounding neurology (neuro-hospitalist or stroke physician), neuroradiology, neurosurgery, nursing and physical medicine and rehabilitation.

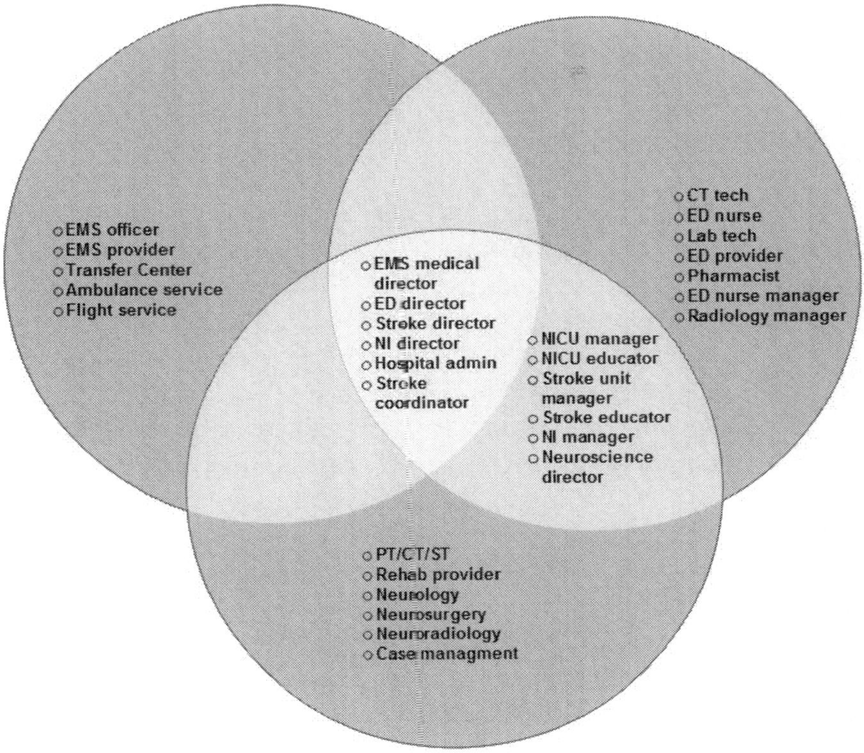

Figure 7.1. Chart showing all different disciplines in stroke teams. Core stroke team includes leaders from all three different teams.

Like any large team, the stroke team needs written protocols to guide its operation, regulate work flow, and determine accountability. The protocols must outline responsibilities of each member and help with setting goals that need to be accomplished. Simple and well-thought of flow charts should be built to reflect protocols. They should be posted in all areas of stroke care. Representatives from each discipline should participate with creating and designing these protocols. Protocols should be reviewed and revised annually and should be reflective of the latest AHA/ASA guidelines.

▪ Proposed protocols

EMS field triage protocol

EMS personnel field protocols should be very simple and straightforward to guarantee fast assessment and triage. The basic steps of field triaging process using FAST scale and any of the LVO scales discussed in chapter 5 is shown in Figure 7.2.

This algorithm needs to be customized based on geographic location and capability of hospitals in the area. Stroke leaders should develop enough knowledge about each hospitals' capabilities before making the protocol. EMS's main task by order is 1) to stabilize the patient; 2) to determine if stroke is a high possibility or not; 3) to determine if there is likelihood of large vessel occlusion (LVO, by using standardized regional LVO scale); (4) to determine the best available stroke center for a particular patient in certain geographic location (as determined by pre-set protocols); 5) to send acute standardized notification to receiving team and to deliver the patient as quickly as possible based on weather and other logistical considerations.

Stroke code team protocol

Algorithm in figure 7.3 is designed to be a simple guide that may be customized based on stroke level designation of the receiving hospital and background of stroke team members.

The process starts with receiving notification from emergency room team and preferably from EMS personnel directly from the field. Stroke team including ED stroke treating

Figure 7.2. Emergency service stroke triage algorithm.

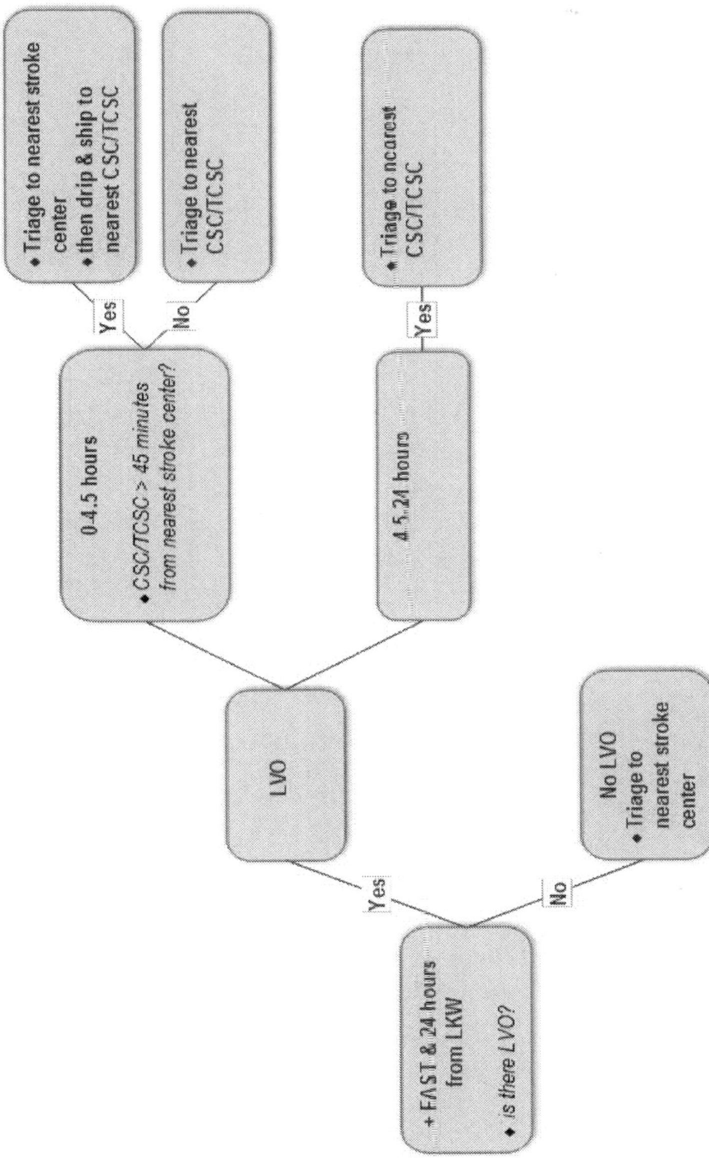

team (nurse/physician), CT technologists, ECG technologist, X-ray technologist, stroke/neurology team (if available) should meet the patient in the CT suite. Stroke code team may include critical care stroke nurse who will admit the patient after IV tPA and/or EVT.

ED treating team should perform a very quick assessment to ensure patient stability and confirm neurological findings (NIHSS) without delaying CT scan. If patient arrives without IV access, treating team should obtain an 18-gauge IV access immediately after obtaining head NCCT.

This protocol should be posted in ED department, NICU, stroke unit and CT suite to guide team members.

Severe ischemic strokes (LVO) that present to ASRH or PSC might pose a challenge to ED and stroke team. They have to be prepared to give IV tPA to appropriate candidate patient, communicate with the local neurologist over the phone or through tele medicine system (in case of ARSH) and at the same time they should have open communication with nearest CSC or TCSC and an accepting NI physician to arrange patient transfer immediately after IV tPA is started. Transferring patient is not an easy task especially when transferring agency is a third party.

It is not uncommon that transfers take tremendous amount of time. Actually, transfer delay is considered one of the significant factors limiting the use of EVT in acute ischemic stroke. A study published in 2001 showed that the likelihood of receiving EVT decreases rapidly by increasing transfer time. In this study, the median hospital-to-hospital distance was 14.7 miles and median transfer time was 104 minutes. Transfer time was 33% lower among those who underwent emergent angiography. The odds of treatment decrease by 2.5% for every minute of transfer time [(1)].

Despite lack of enough research to make robust recommendations regarding where patients with severe stroke symptoms (LVO) should be triaged to initially, based on this study and author's experience, if nearest CSC or TCSC is more 45 minutes away from the nearest hospital, patient should be triaged directly to CSC/TCSC.

In a different study, large volume centers were faster with giving IV tPA than medium and small volume centers. Patients admitted to hospitals with an annual thrombolysis volume of ≥50 cases per annum had median arrival-tPA times that were 28 and 22 minutes shorter than patients admitted to hospitals with volumes of 0 to 24 and 25 to 49, respectively. Onset-tPA times were shorter by 24 to 32 minutes across strata of onset-arrival times. In multivariable analysis, patients admitted to hospitals with a volume of ≥50 cases per annum had 4.33 the odds of receiving tPA within 60 minutes of arrival. No differences in safety outcomes were observed, with similar 30-day mortality and complication rates across the groups [(2)]. Regional stroke leaders should keep this data in mind when designing regional stroke triaging protocols.

ED ICH and SAH protocol

Stroke code and ED teams should work together on stabilizing ICH and SAH patients immediately after diagnosis recognition on head NCCT. As with acute ischemic stroke, it is imperative to recognize both ICH and SAH as a condition that requires immediate attention and intervention to stabilize BP and reverse anticoagulation. Obtaining emergent consultation from specialized team is equally critical. Figure 7.4 provides a stabilization guide until the patient care is taken over by a more specialized team.

Figure 7.3. Emergency room stroke work-up algorithm.

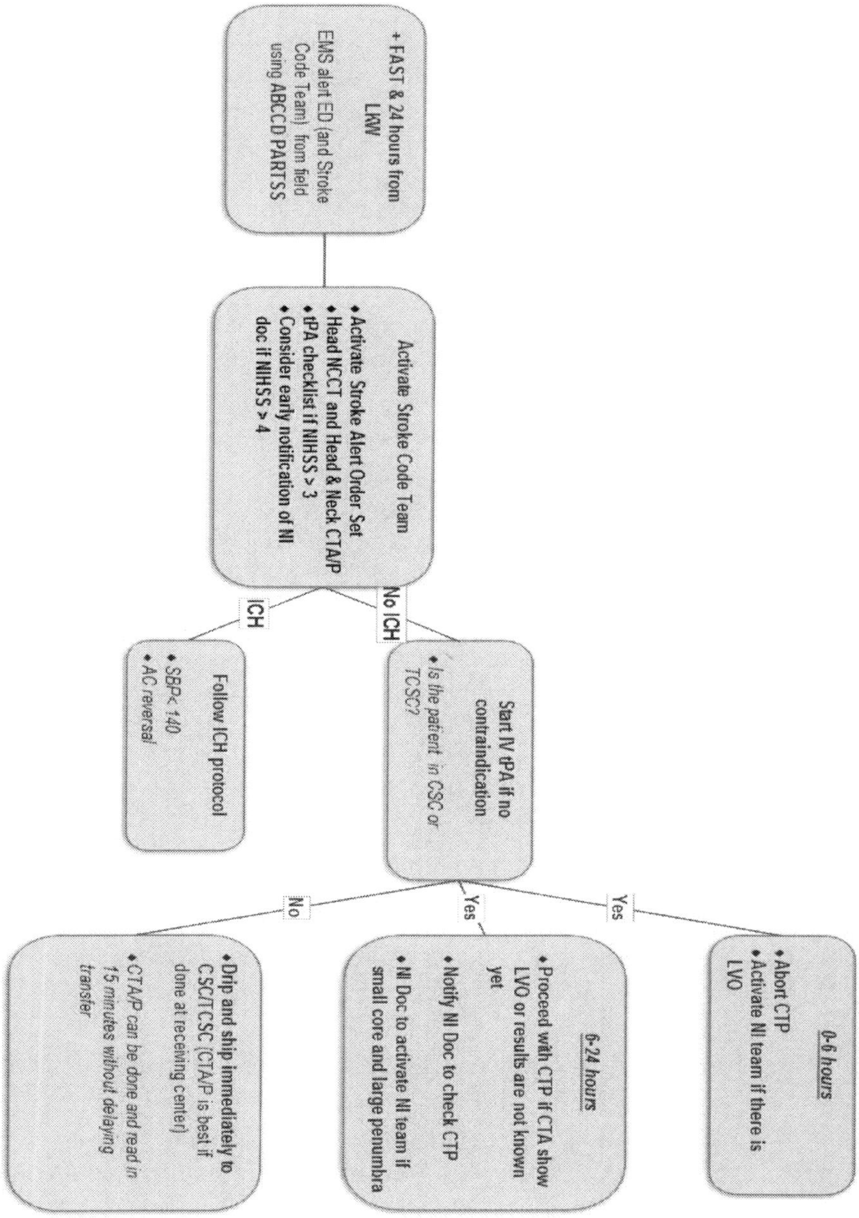

Figure 7.4. Emergency room ICH/SAH work-up algorithm.

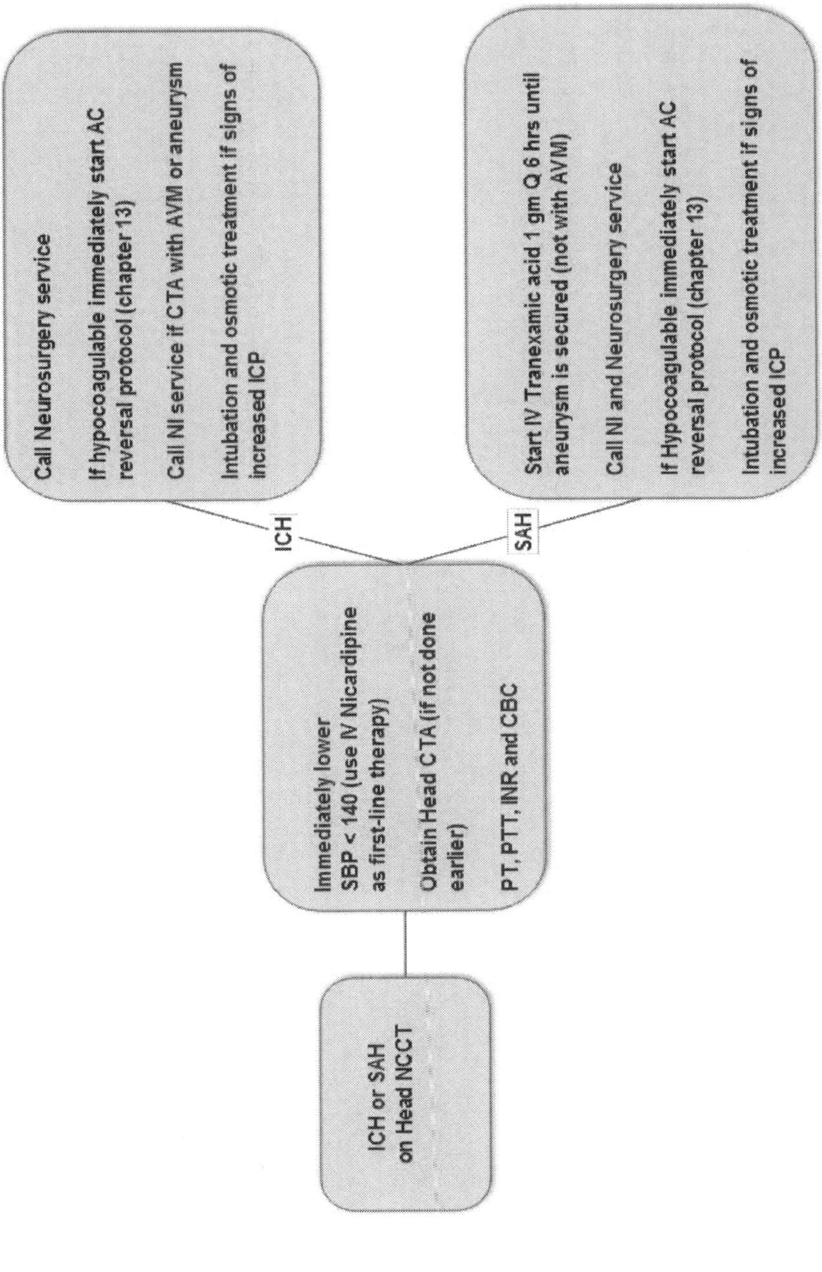

References

1. *Transfer delay is a major factor limiting the use of intra-arterial treatment in acute ischemic stroke* . Prabhakaran S, Ward E, John S. 6, s.l. : Stroke, 2011, Vol. 42.
2. *Bigger, faster? Associations between hospital thrombolysis volume and speed of thrombolysis administration in acute ischemic stroke.* Bray BD, Campbell J, Cloud GC. 11, s.l. : Stroke, 2013, Vol. 44.

8

Endovascular Treatment of Ischemic Stroke

▪ Endovascular treatment

Early recanalization of occluded vessels in acute ischemic stroke (AIS) either by IV tPA or endovascular revascularization has been shown to be associated with improved clinical outcome and reduced mortality. Initial data on endovascular treatment (EVT) of AIS was published in the 1980s. Since then, endovascular techniques for AIS treatment tremendously improved, advancing from intra-arterial administration of thrombolytic drugs to first-generation mechanical thrombectomy devices (Merci clot retriever and Penumbra clot aspiration) and more recently to second-generation mechanical thrombectomy devices (stent-retrievers) [(1)] (Figure 8.1).

First Generation (Table 8.1)

In 2004, the Merci retriever (Concentric Medical, Mountain View, CA) was the first device approved for removal of thrombus from intracranial arteries by the Food and Drug Administration (FDA) [(1)].

In 2008, the Penumbra clot aspiration system (Penumbra, Inc, Alameda, CA) was the second device for AIS that was approved by the FDA. This device enables a thrombus aspiration by use of a large lumen catheter positioned in contact with the clot and attached to a vacuum pump [1] (Figure 8.3).

Table 8.1. Trials of first-generation clot retrievers.

Studies on First Generation of Clot Retrievers [1]						
Study	**Devices**	**Patients**	**TIMI II/III %**	**mRS ≤ 2 %**	**Hemorrhage %**	**Mortality %**
MERCI	Merci	151	46	25	7.8	43.5
Multi-MERCI	Merci	177	68	36	9.8	34
Penumbra	Penumbra	125	81.6	25	11.2	32
Penumbra-POST	Penumbra	157	87	41	6.4	20

Second Generation (Table 8.2)

Traditional detachable stents are designed to be detached in the vasculature after being delivered in the target vessel. On the other hand, nondetachable neurovascular stents (2nd generation stents) are proven to be more useful with foreign body and clot removal (in-vitro and in-vivo studies) due to that fact that nondetachable stents (including stent-retrievers) can be temporarily placed in the vasculature but removed after use. Because of its frequent and successful off-label use, the nondetachable Solitaire intracranial stent (Covidien/EV3; Plymouth, MN) turned into a primary clot retriever [1].

Table 8.2. Trials of second-generation clot retrievers.

Studies on Second Generation of Clot Retrievers [1]				
Study	**Devices**	**Patients**	**IV tPA**	**Recanalization %**
SWIFT	Solitaire	58	33	61
STAR	Solitaire	202	59	79.2
TREVO	TREVO	60	60	91.7
TREVO 2	TREVO	88	58	92
NASA registry	Solitaire	354	45	87.5

Stent-retrievers combine two mechanisms of action: 1) the deployment of the stent-retriever within the clot immediately restores blood flow and 2) the mesh of stent-retriever embedded within the clot serves to catch and retrieve the clot (Figure 8.3). Though most clots are successfully retrieved after one to two passes, several passes with the stent-retriever to the occluded site through a microcatheter are infrequently necessary [1]. Also, combining aspiration with the clot retriever showed higher recanalization rates than the use of each technology alone.

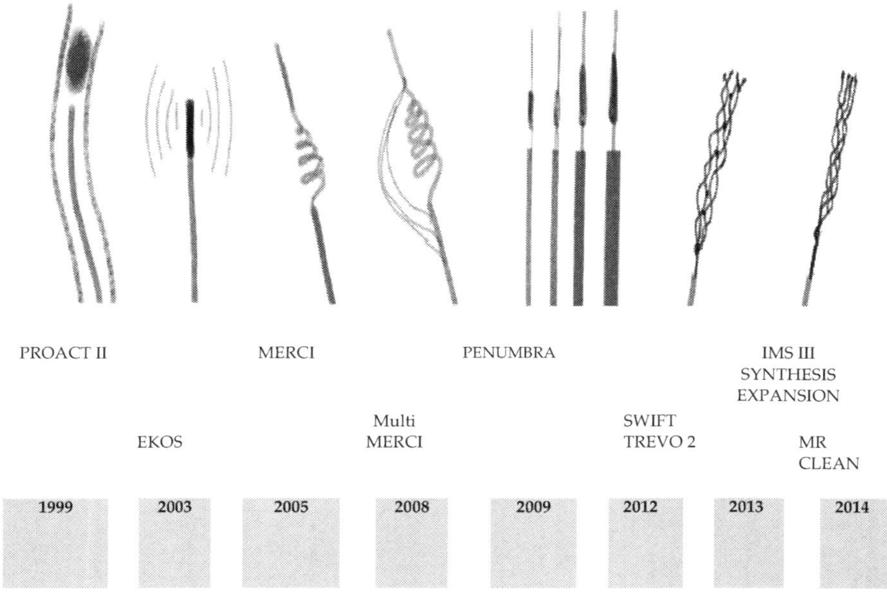

Figure 8.1. Mechanical clot removal devices evolution with respective clinical trials.

▪ Clinical trials

EVT of stroke and supporting evidence evolved relatively quickly over the last decade (Figure 8.1). The following is an overview of most significant clinical stroke interventional trials. These trials mainly tested anterior circulation strokes. They used modified Rankin Scale (mRS) as a clinical outcome measure, the same scale used to measure IV tPA outcome in the NINDs trial (Table 8.3). Overall, scale 0-3 is considered good outcome [(2)]. These trials used mainly aspiration and stent-retriever techniques (Figure 8.2 and 8.3).

Table 8.3. modified Rankin Scale (mRS).

modified Rankin Scale (mRS)	
0	No symptoms at all
1	No disability despite symptoms; able to carry out all usual duties
2	Slight disability; unable to perform all previous activities, but able to look after own affairs without assistance
3	Moderate disability; requiring some help, but able to walk without assistance
4	Moderately severe disability; unable to walk or attend to own bodily needs without assistance
5	Severe disability; bedridden, incontinent and requiring constant nursing care & attention
6	Death

Table. 8.4. Cerebral recanalization scale.

Thrombolysis in Cerebral Infarction (TICI)	
0	No perfusion
1	Penetration, but no distal branch filling
2a	Perfusion with incomplete (<50%) distal branch filling
2b	Perfusion with incomplete (>50%) distal branch filling
3	Full perfusion with filling of all distal branches

The trial also included angiographic result as an outcome and used Thrombolysis in Cerebral Infarction (TICI) (Figure 8.4 and Table 8.4). Overall TICI 2b and 3 correlates with good outcome. Mainly mortality and symptomatic ICH were measured complications. Symptomatic hemorrhage is any hemorrhagic transformation temporally related to any worsening in neurological condition.

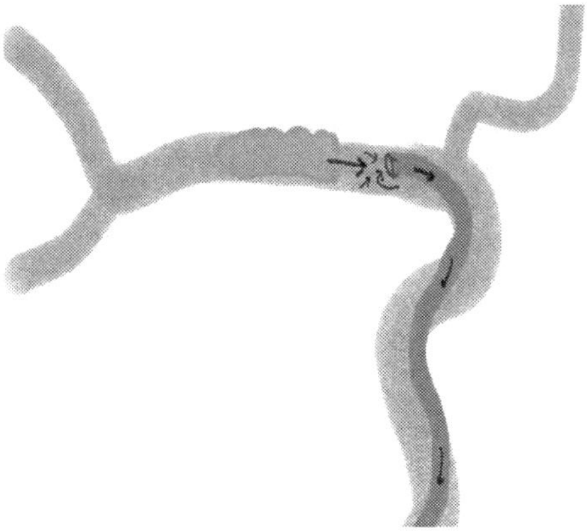

Figure 8.2. Aspiration catheter used to aspirate the clot from its proximal to distal end. Negative pressure is produced by a pump attached to proximal end of the catheter.

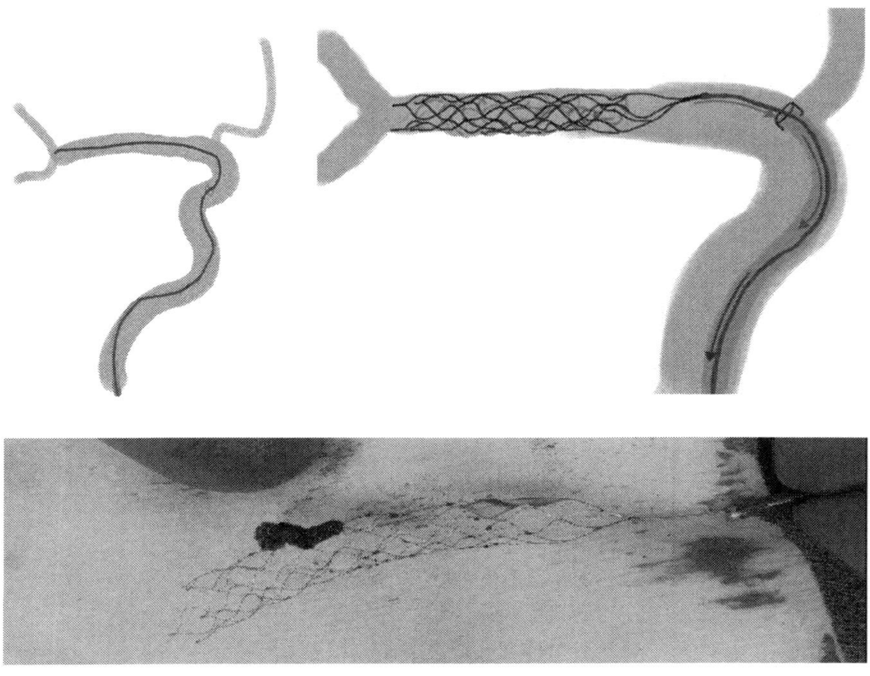

Figure 8.3. Stent-retriever used to retrieve MCA clot. First, microcatheter used to cross clot; then the stent-retriever is deployed in the clot and is pulled outside while open.

IMS 3 (3)

This is a multicenter, randomized, open-label trial.

- Patients: 656 adult (age 18-82) patients received IV tPA within 3 hours of onset and had NIHSS 10 or more (NIHSS 10 is considered severe stroke due to major arterial occlusion).
- Intervention: IV tPA (⅔ usual dose) plus EVT (approach chosen by the interventionalist).
- Comparison: IV tPA alone (usual dose).
- Primary outcome: mRS of 2 or less at 90 days.

Results

- There was no difference in the primary outcome (mRS <3): 40.8% with EVT and 38.7% with IV tPA alone.
- No difference in mortality (19.1% vs 21.6%).
- No difference in symptomatic ICH (sICH, 6.2% vs 5.9%). There was an increase in asymptomatic ICH with EVT (27.4% vs 18.9%).

Comments

- The trial was stopped early for futility.
- The trial initially used the NIHSS score to identify major arterial occlusion, although it is only 80% accurate. As the trial progressed, more centers starting using CT angiography.

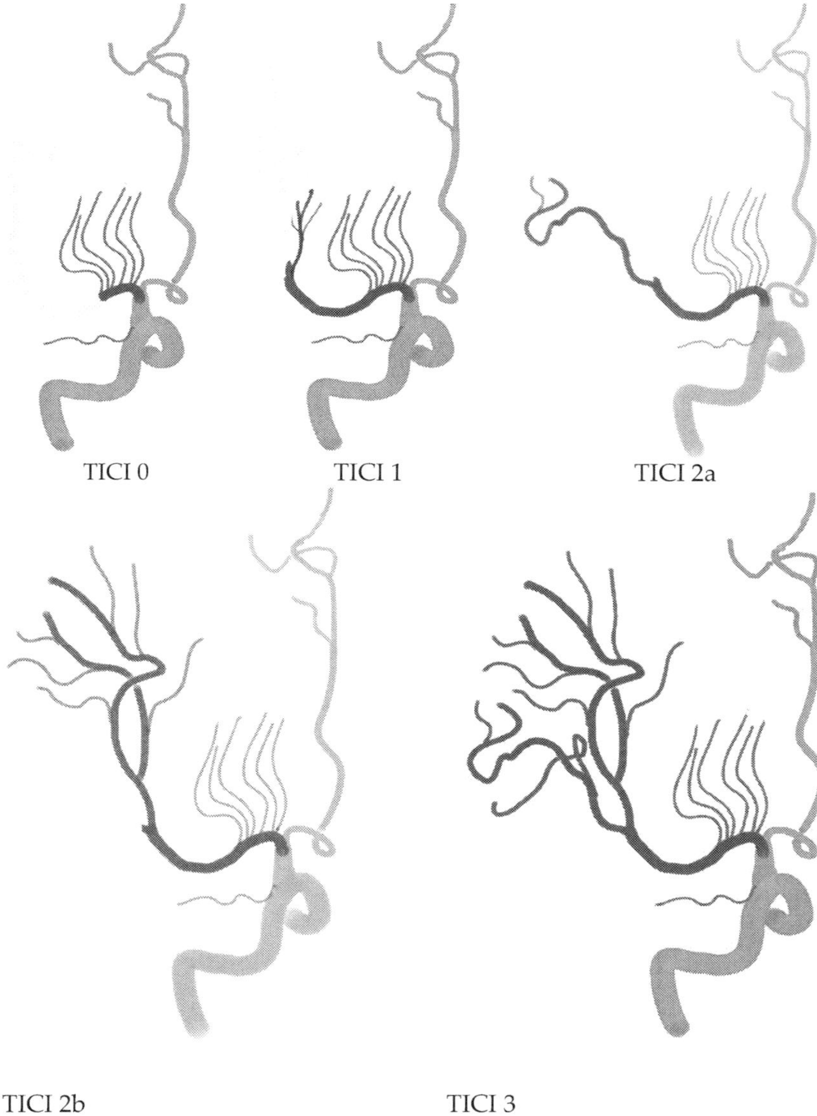

Figure 8.4. Thrombolysis in Cerebral Infarction (TICI). See Table 8.4. for description.

SYNTHESIS [4]

This is a pragmatic, multicenter, randomized, open-label trial.

- Patients: 362 adult (age 18-80) ischemic stroke patients within 4.5 hours of symptom onset if receiving IV tPA or 6 hours for interventions.
- Intervention: EVT (no IV tPA) (mostly intra-arterial tPA, about ⅓ had a device used).
- Comparison: IV tPA.
- Primary outcome: Disability free survival (mRS 0-1) at 90 days.

Results

- The primary outcome (disability free survival, mRS 0-1, at 90 days) was the same in both groups: 30.4% with EVT and 34.8% with standard care.
- No difference in mortality: 8% with EVT and 6% with IV tPA.
- No difference in sICH, 6% vs 6%.

Comments

- EVT took about 1 hour longer to get started than tPA.
- Accepting different times for the different groups might be problematic.
- The patients treated earlier have better outcomes and are over-represented in the earlier time frames.
- Primary outcome collected by telephone.

MR RESCUE (5)

This is a phase 2, multicenter, randomized, open-label trial.

- Patients: 118 adult (age 18-85) patients within 8 hours of large vessel, anterior-circulation strokes. Patients were all treated with IV tPA and were eligible if there was no recanalization on a subsequent CT or MR angiogram.
- Intervention: mechanical embolectomy.
- Comparison: standard care.
- Primary outcome: mRS at 90 days.

Results

- Same mean score on the mRS at 90 days (3.9 vs 3.9).
- 17 (24%) patients in the EVT had complications.
- 90 days mortality was very high (21%) and not different between groups.

Comments

- This is an exceptionally select subgroup. 127 patients from 22 centers over 7 years means each center contribute less than one patient per year.

MR CLEAN (6)

This is randomized clinical trial with open-label treatment and blinded end-point evaluation.

- Patients: 500 adult (18 years and older) patients. EVT was offered within 6 hours of symptom onset. It included anterior circulation stroke (distal internal carotid, middle cerebral artery, or anterior cerebral artery) based on CTA or MRA.

- Intervention: intra-arterial treatment at the discretion of the treating physician (mechanical, intra-arterial thrombolysis, or both).
- Comparison: usual care
- Primary outcome: mRS at 90 days (collected by telephone interview).

Results

- Improved excellent outcome (mRS 0-1): 11.6% vs 6.0%.
- Improved functional independence (mRS 0-2): 32.6% vs 19.1%.
- No difference in 30-day mortality: 18.9% vs 18.4%
- No difference in sICH: 7.7% vs 6.4%

Comments

- 89% of patients received IV tPA.
- 84% of the EVT group had some kind of intra-arterial therapy done.
- 30 patients in the EVT arm also had stenting of their internal carotid done at the time of the procedure.
- There was an absolute difference of 13.5 % points in the rate of functional independence (mRS, 0 to 2) in favor of the intervention (32.6% vs. 19.1%).
- There were no significant differences in mortality or the occurrence of sICH.

EXTEND IA [7]

This is a multicenter, randomized, open-label trial.

- Patients: 70 adult patients received IV tPA within 4.5 hours of symptom onset. It included internal carotid or middle cerebral artery and evidence of salvageable brain tissue on CT perfusion (CTP).
- Intervention: IV tPA plus EVT initiated within 6 hours.
- Comparison: IV tPA alone.
- Primary outcome: Co-primary outcomes were reperfusion at 24 hours and early neurologic improvement (≥8-point reduction on the NIHSS or a score of 0 or 1 at day 3).

Results

- More reperfusion at 24 hours (100% vs. 37%).
- Increased neurologic improvement at 3 days (80% vs. 37%).
- Improved functional independence (mRS 0-2) (71% vs. 40%).
- Non-significant increase in excellent outcome (mRS 0-1) (51% vs 29%).
- No difference in mortality. EVT group did better (9% vs 20%).
- No difference in sICH (2 vs 0 patients).

Comments

- This is a very select group of patients. Only 70 patients enrolled (2.5 patients per center per year).
- Outcome collected was reperfusion, not a patient-oriented outcome.

- Trial was stopped early (original target was 100 patients) based on the MR CLEAN results.

ESCAPE [8]

This is a multicenter, randomized, open-label trial.

- Patients: 316 adult patients (NIHSS>5) within 12 hours after symptom onset. Patients had to have a small infarct core (ASPECTS score 6-10) and a CTA had to demonstrate proximal MCA occlusion, and good collateral circulation (> 50% filling of MCA territory).
- Intervention: EVT in addition to standard care (including IV tPA). (Retrievable stents were recommended).
- Comparison: standard care.
- Primary outcome: mRS at 90 days.

Results

- Increase in functional independence (mRS 0-2): 53.0%, vs. 29.3%.
- Reduced mortality: 10.4%, vs. 19.0%.
- No change in sICH: 3.6% vs 2.7% in the control group.

Comments

- The trial was stopped early. Originally planned to include 500 patients. They had crossed a prespecified boundary for stopping early.
- Very select group of patients.
- Of the patients randomized to EVT, 91.5% actually had EVT.

SWIFT PRIME [9]

This is a multicenter, randomized, open-label trial.

- Patients: 196 adult patients receiving tPA who could get EVT within 6 hours. Patients all had imagining confirmed occlusions in the proximal anterior intracranial circulation and lacked large ischemic cores.
- Intervention: EVT with a stent retriever in addition to tPA.
- Comparison: tPA alone.
- Primary outcome: mRS at 90 days.

Results

- Functional independence (mRS 0-2) was higher in the EVT group: 60% vs 35%.
- There was no difference in mortality (9% vs 12%).

Comments

- The trial was stopped early for efficacy.
- Very select group of patients.
- Imaging criteria was modified halfway into the trial.

REVASCAT [10]

This is a multicenter, randomized, open-label trial.

- Patients: 206 adult ischemic stroke patients within 8 hours. Imaging confirming anterior circulation occlusion without large infarct size. Patients were either ineligible for tPA or had tPA but did not recanalize within 30 minutes. (did not use perfusion imaging as an inclusion criterion).

- Intervention: EVT with the Solitaire stent retriever in addition to medical management (include tPA for eligible patients).
- Comparison: medical management alone.
- Primary outcome: mRS at 90 days.

Results

- Higher rate of functional independence (mRS 0-2) with EVT: 43.7%, 28.2%.
- Mortality non-statistically different (18.4% with EVT vs 15.5%).

Comments

- The trial was stopped early "because of a loss of equipoise" after other trials were published.

DIFFUSE 3 (11)

This is multicenter, randomized, open-label trial, with blinded outcome assessment.

- Patients: 182 patients (92 to EVT group and 90 to medical-therapy group). Treatment was offered 6 to 16 hours after LKW. It included proximal middle cerebral artery or internal carotid artery occlusion, an initial infarct size of less than 70 ml, and a ratio of the volume of ischemic tissue on perfusion imaging to infarct volume of 1.8 or more.
- Intervention: thrombectomy (thrombectomy was performed with any FDA-approved thrombectomy device,

at the discretion of the neurointerventionalist) plus standard medical therapy.

- Comparison: standard medical therapy alone.
- Primary outcome: mRS at 90 days.

Results

- Higher percentage of patients who were functionally independent; mRS of 0 to 2 (45%, 17%).
- No difference in mortality rate was (14, 26%).
- No difference in sICH (7%, 4%) or serious adverse events (43%, 53%).

Comments:

- The power to assess the response to therapy in subgroups was limited due to the lower than anticipated number of patients enrolled as a result of early termination of the trial.

DAWN (12)

This is multicenter, randomized, open-label trial.

- Patients: 206 patients (107 to EVT group and 99 to the medical therapy group). Treatment was offered 6 to 24 hours after LKW if it included proximal middle cerebral artery or internal carotid artery occlusion. Mismatch between the severity of the clinical deficit and the infarct volume, with mismatch criteria defined according to age (<80 years or ≥80 years).

- Intervention: EVT (thrombectomy using Trevo device; Stryker Neurovascular) plus standard medical therapy.
- Comparison: standard medical therapy alone.
- Primary outcome: mRS at 90 days.

Results

- Higher percentage of patients were functionally independent; mRS 0-2 (49%, 13%).
- No difference in mortality rate was (19, 18%).
- No significant difference in sICH (6%, 3%).

Comments:

- Randomization was stratified according to prognostic variables that the investigators determined to be most pertinent in the patient population.

Summary

It is very obvious that these trials answered the big question regarding efficacy of EVT in AIS. Actually, EVT is one of the most powerful treatment tools in modern medicine. However, there is still another major question: "what is the best triaging protocol?" which is still not completely resolved.

References:

1. *Techniques for Endovascular Treatment of Acute Ischemic Stroke From Intra-Arterial Fibrinolytics to Stent-Retrievers.* Laurent Pierot, Sébastien Soize , Azzedine Benaissa. s.l. : Stroke, 2015, Vol. 46.
2. Morgenstern, Justin. *Interventional therapy for acute ischemic stroke: the evidence.* [Online] July 11, 2017. https://first10em.com/interventional-therapy-stroke/.
3. *Endovascular therapy after intravenous t-PA versus t-PA alone for stroke.* Broderick JP, Palesch YY, Demchuk AM. 10, s.l. : The New England Journal of Medicine, 2013, Vol. 368.
4. *Endovascular treatment for acute ischemic stroke.* Ciccone A, Valvassori L, Nichelatti M. 10, s.l. : The New England Journal of Medicine, 2013, Vol. 368.
5. *A trial of imaging selection and endovascular treatment for ischemic stroke.* Kidwell CS, Jahan R, Gornbein J. 10, s.l. : The New England Journal of Medicine, 2013, Vol. 368.
6. *A randomized trial of intraarterial treatment for acute ischemic stroke.* Berkhemer OA, Fransen PS, Beumer D. 1, s.l. : The New England Journal of Medicine, 2015, Vol. 372.
7. *Endovascular therapy for ischemic stroke with perfusion-imaging selection.* Campbell BC, Mitchell PJ, Kleinig TJ. 11, s.l. : The New England Journal of Medicine, 2015, Vol. 372.
8. *Randomized assessment of rapid endovascular treatment of ischemic stroke.* Goyal M, Demchuk AM, Menon BK. 11, s.l. : The New England Journal of Medicine, 2015, Vol. 372.
9. *Stent-retriever thrombectomy after intravenous t-PA vs. t-PA alone in stroke.* Saver JL, Goyal M, Bonafe A. 24, s.l. : The New England Journal of Medicine, 2015, Vol. 372.
10. *Thrombectomy within 8 hours after symptom onset in ischemic stroke.* Jovin TG, Chamorro A, Cobo E. 24, s.l. : The New England Journal of Medicine, 2015, Vol. 372.
11. *Thrombectomy for Stroke at 6 to 16 Hours with Selection by Perfusion Imaging.* G.W. Albers, M.P. Marks, S. Kemp, S. 8, s.l. : The new england journal of medicine, 2018, Vol. 378.
12. *Thrombectomy 6 to 24 Hours after Stroke with a Mismatch between Deficit and Infarct.* Raul G. Nogueira, M.D., Ashutosh P. Jadhav, M.D., Ph.D., Diogo C. Haussen, M.D. 11, s.l. : The New England Journal of Medicine, Vol. 378.

9

Stroke Imaging

The main role of acute stroke imaging studies is to exclude hemorrhage, to assess the extent of brain injury, and to identify the vascular lesion causing the ischemia. Some advanced CT and MRI technologies are able to distinguish between dead brain tissue (core) and that which is potentially salvageable (penumbra). This aids the treating team in selecting patients likely to benefit from acute interventional stroke therapy [(1)].

▪ Non-contract CT (NCCT)

The main reason why head NCCT is first line imaging modality in acute stroke is that CTs are widely available and very fast to acquire and process. In the hyperacute phase, NCCT scan is obtained to mainly exclude or confirm intracerebral hemorrhage (ICH). It is highly sensitive for this indication. Immediate CT scanning of all patients with suspected stroke is also the most cost-effective strategy when compared with alternate strategies such as scanning select patients or delayed rather than immediate imaging. NCCT for brain ischemia sensitivity is greatest after 24 hours. However, the prevalence of early CT signs of brain infarction is 61 % within 6 hours of stroke onset [(2)].

Typical appearance of ischemic stroke on NCCT is a hypodensity (Figure 9.1a). The hypodensity appearance is due to cytotoxic edema (irreversible damage) and might not be visible until 12-24 hours after stroke onset. Hypodensity is not only seen in ischemic stroke, but also with venous stroke secondary to CVT and with vasogenic edema due to tumor or infection.

On the other hand, bleed appears as a hyperdensity due to dense appearance of blood (Figure 9.1b). Hyperdensity can also be due to calcifications found in AVMs, calcified aneurysms, calcified tumors, and atherosclerosis.

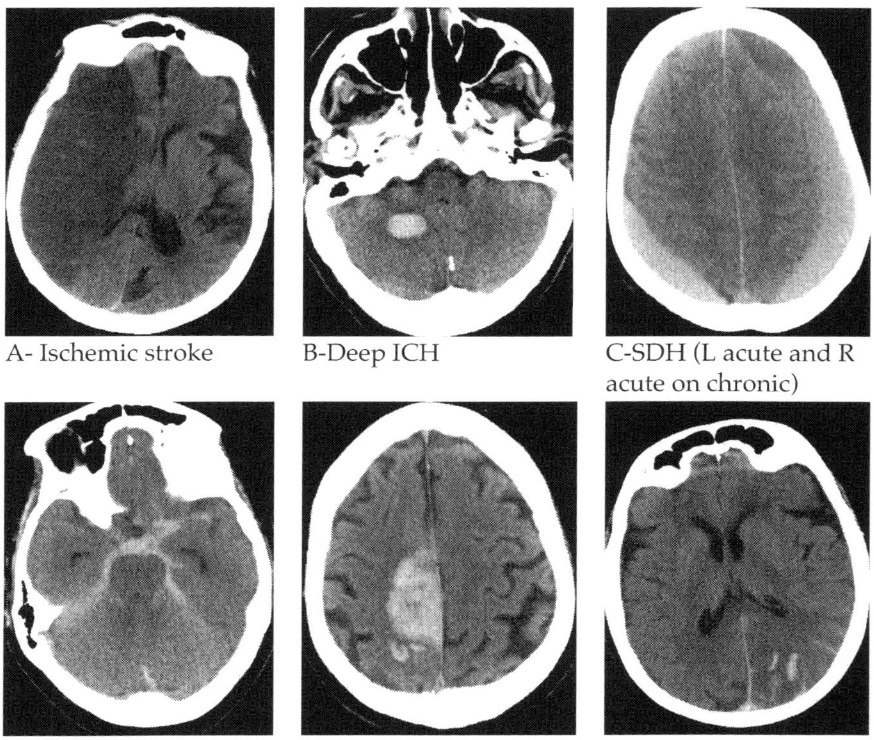

A- Ischemic stroke | B-Deep ICH | C-SDH (L acute and R acute on chronic)

D- SAH | D-Lobar ICH | E- Venous infarction

Figure 9.1. NCCT images for ischemic stroke (A); Deep ICH (B); SDH (C); Subarachnoid hemorrhage, SAH (D); Lobar ICH (D); CVT with resultant venous stroke and ICH (E).

Early signs of ischemia

In ischemic stroke, NCCT can detect edematous changes secondary to cytotoxic edema due to the failure of ion pumps. A decreased attenuation of water in the brain will locally result in lower Hounsfield Units (darker area) [3] [4]:

1. *Hypoattenuation of basal ganglia and the middle cerebral artery territory*

Hypoattenuation, especially in the basal ganglia, is an early ischemic stroke. Hypoattenuation can be detected within 6 hours after stroke onset. If hypoattenuation is mainly described in middle cerebral artery (MCA) territory, the basal ganglia is frequently involved. It is also important to assess stroke volume using semi-quantitative scoring system to determine whether less or more than one-third of the MCA flow territory is involved.

There are other terms to describe early ischemic changes (Figure 9.2):

1. Obscuration of lentiform nucleus that is detected within 2 hours.
2. Loss of gray-white matter differentiation in the basal ganglia.
3. Cortical sulcal effacement where the delineation between gray and white matter becomes less clear due to mass effect.
4. The loss of insular ribbon and obscuration of Sylvian fissure sign where there is fading of the discrete delineation of the gray-white matter interface at the lateral margin of the insula.
5. The "dense artery sign" which is hyper-attenuation (brightness) of a brain vessel due to intravascular clot formation in the artery. This is easier to notice in MCA. Dense sign can be enhanced by thin-section NCCT imaging with maximal intensity projection (MIP) reconstruction [5].

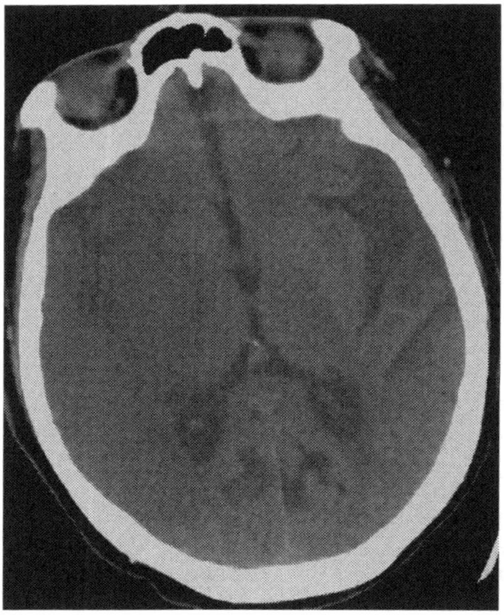

Loss of grey white differentiation in basal ganglia, loss of insular ribbon and obscuration of Sylvian fissure.

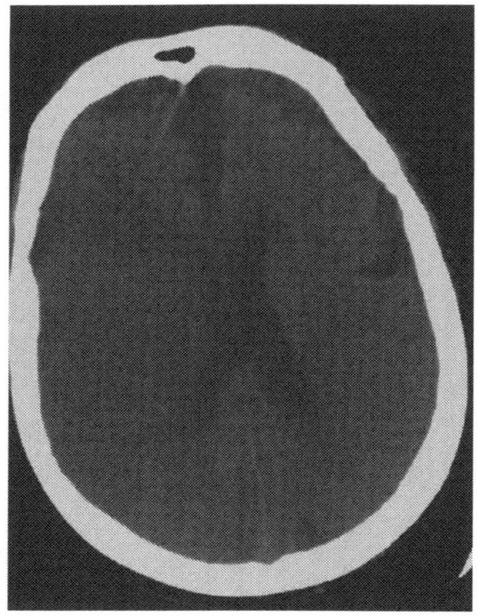

Cortical sulcal effacement.

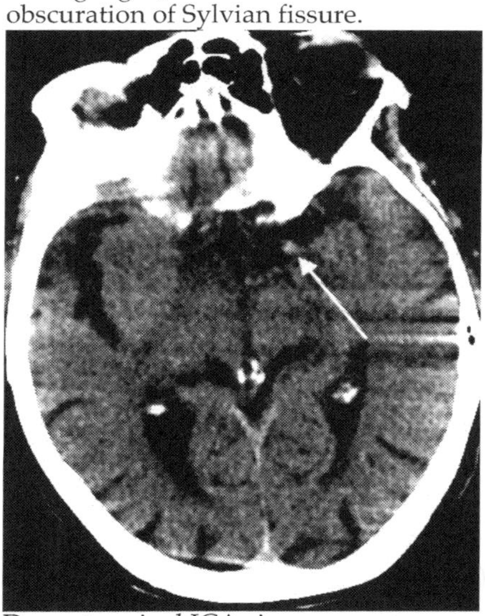

Dense terminal ICA sign

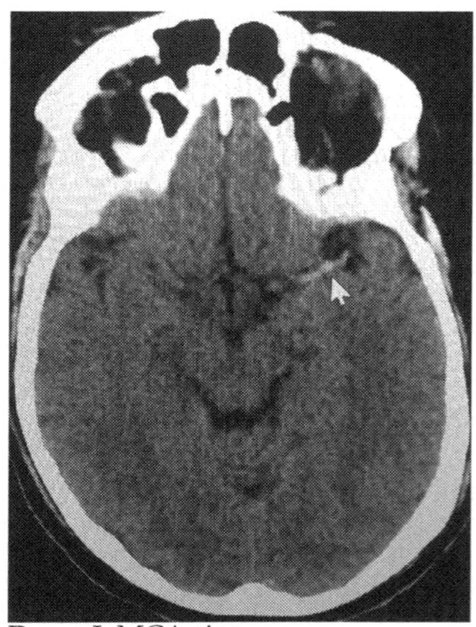

Dense L MCA sign

Figure 9.2. NCCT showing early ischemic changes.

2. *The ASPECT Score*

ASPECT (Alberta Stroke Program Early CT) score is a tool to analyze hypoattenuation in different brain regions (Figure 9.3). The ASPECT score is a number between 1 and 10 based on the number of affected brain regions. ASPECT score can be used for prognostication and indications for treatment. The lower the score, the worse the expected outcome [6].

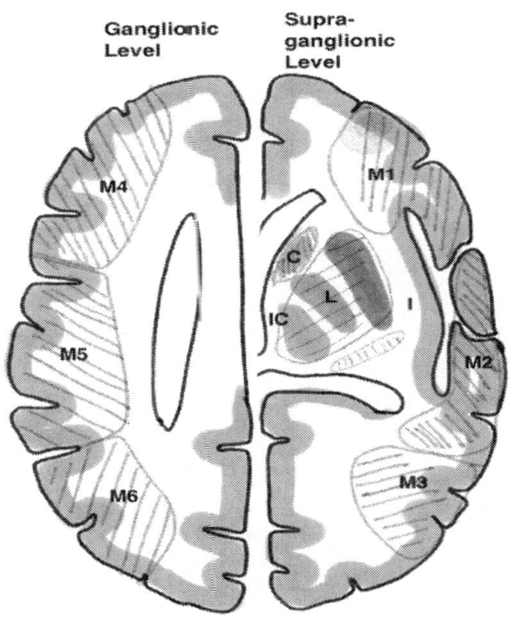

Figure 9.3. **ASPECT score**. **C**- Caudate, **I**- Insular ribbon, **IC**- Internal Capsule, **L**- Lentiform nucleus, **M1**-Anterior MCA, **M2**-MCA cortex lateral to the insular ribbon, **M3**-Posterior MCA cortex, **M4**- Anterior superior MCA cortex, **M5**- Lateral superior MCA area, **M6**-Posterior superior MCA area.
Small core: 8-10; moderate core: 6-7; large core: 0-5. ASPECT Score = /10.

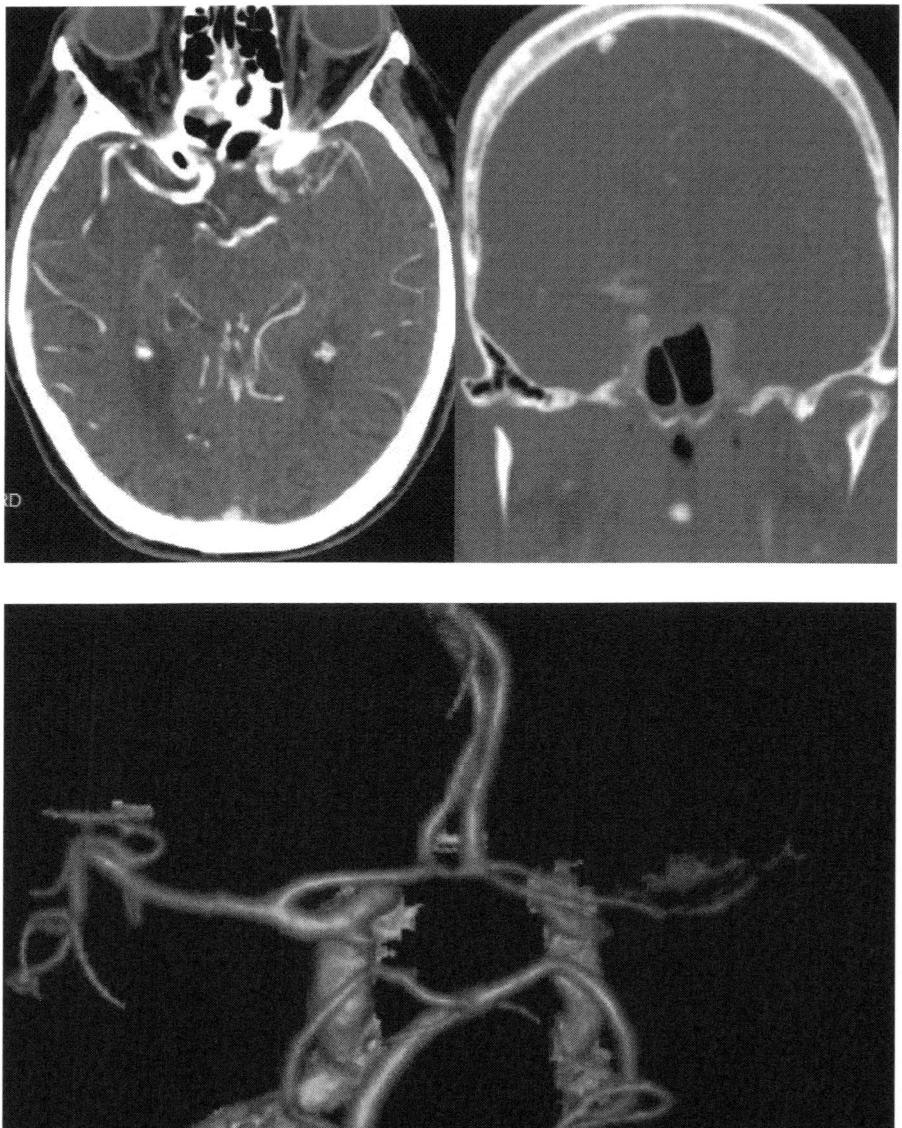

Figure 9.4. Head CTA (axial, coronal and 3D) shows left internal carotid terminus and MCA occlusion (large vessel occlusion; LVO).

▪ Head and neck CT angiogram (CTA)

CTA is the modality of choice to detect large vessel occlusion (LVO) and is usually done immediately following NCCT (Figure 9.4). It is quick, inexpensive, and safe. For the same reason NCCT is first line modality to image the brain, CTA is first line modality to image neck and brain vessels because the time required to perform a CTA is 5 minutes, and the radiation exposure is not significantly high [7].

CTA acquisition requires infusing IV contrast through an 18-gauge IV using a power injector. The cost of performing a CTA in the acute stroke setting is minimal when compared to the costs of untreated stroke. Long-standing concerns surrounding the renal toxicity of CTA contrast appear to be overstated. A large retrospective study found that CTA was associated with transient contrast-induced nephropathy in only 2.9% of patients, none of whom experienced permanent kidney injury or required dialysis [8].

In addition to its tremendous value in detecting LVO in acute ischemic stroke, CTA has many other valuable indications such as extracranial (cervical carotid and vertebral arteries) and intracranial (intracranial carotid artery, MCA, ACA, PCA) atherosclerotic disease, cerebral aneurysms and AVMs, cervical (carotid and vertebral arteries) and cranial arterial dissection, cerebral vasospasm, cerebral venous thrombosis (CVT) and vasculopathies (such CNS vasculitis, drug-induced vasculopathies) (Figure 9.5).

Dual-energy CTA is a newer technology that is preferred for vascular lesions rich with calcium, or when there is metal artifact near the vessel of interest due to nearby aneurysm clip or coil or stent.

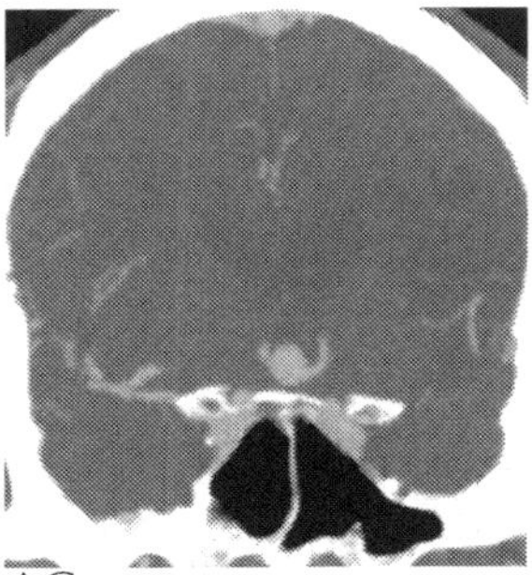

ACom artery aneurysm (coronal view)

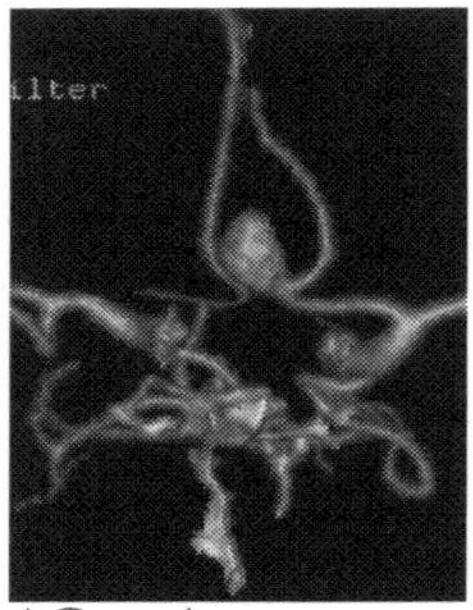

ACom A aneurysm (3D CTA)

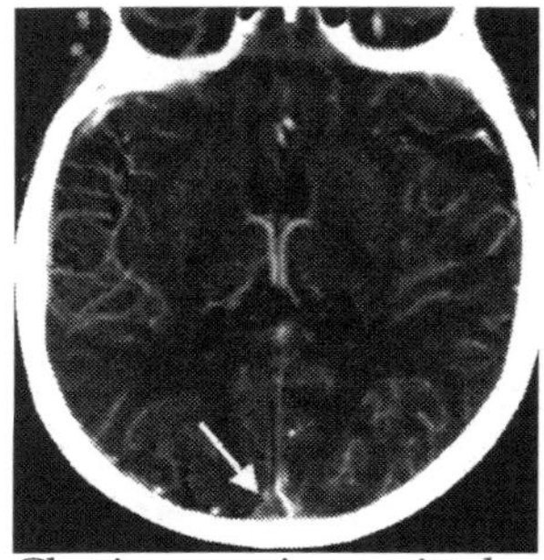

Clot in superior sagittal sinus (delta sign)

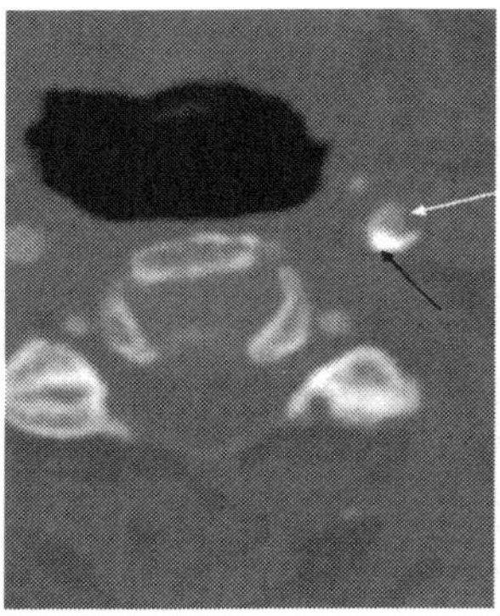

L CCA atherosclerotic stenosis (axial view)

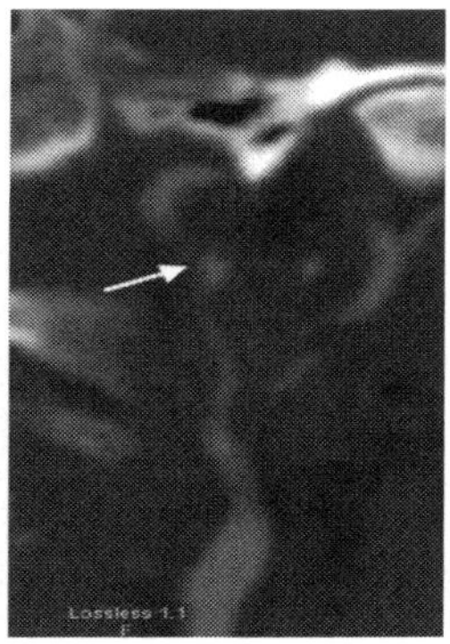

L ICA dissection (diffuse stenosis)

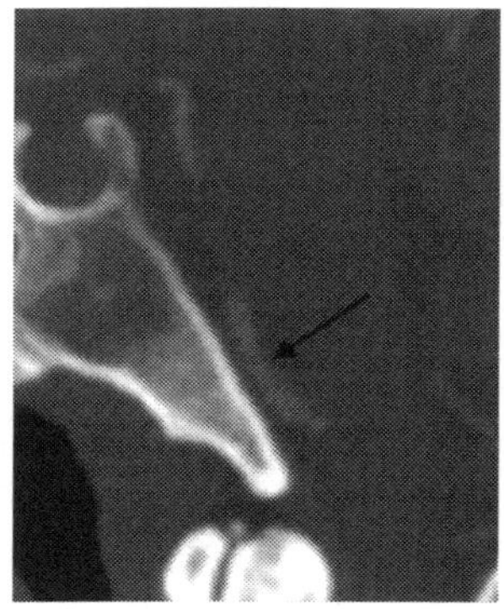

Left VA intracranial stenosis (sagittal view)

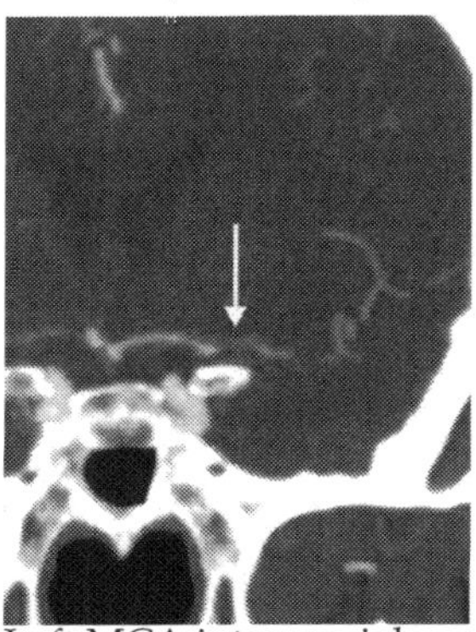

Left MCA intracranial stenosis (coronal view)

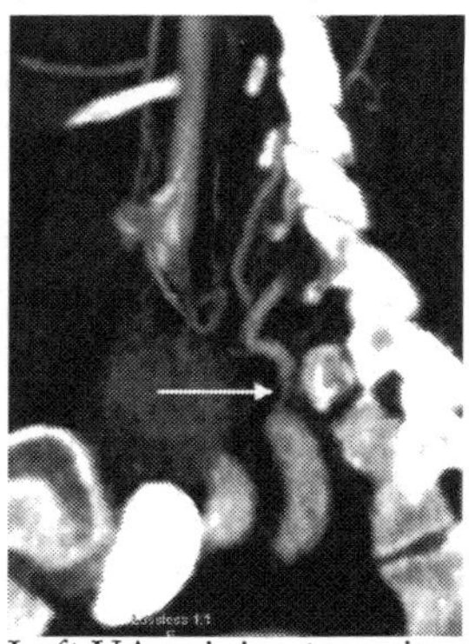

Left VA origin stenosis (sagittal view)

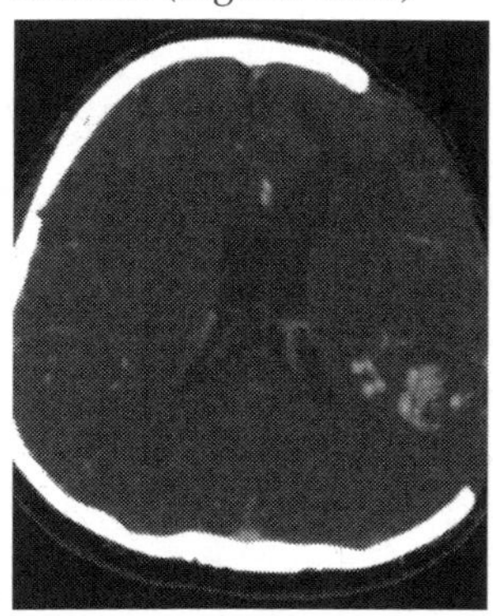

Left temporal AVM (tangle of vessels)

Figure 9.5. Multiple vascular lesions visualized on CTA of head and neck.

▪ Brain CT perfusion (CTP)

Brain CT perfusion (CTP) is an imaging technique that provides quantitative evaluation of cerebral perfusion by generating maps of cerebral blood flow (CBF), cerebral blood volume (CBV), time to maximum residue (Tmax) and mean transit time (MTT) (Figure 9.6). Its main advantage is distinguishing dead area (low CBV) from penumbra (low CBF with normal CBV). Cerebral perfusion CT is fast and available for most standard spiral CT scanners equipped with the appropriate software [9]. Figure 9.7 shows successful example of EVT for the same patient (as Figure 9.6) with a significant penumbra on CTP.

Tmax is the main indicator for ischemia. Tmax value > 6 seconds can estimate tissue that is likely to be critically hypoperfused (CBF <20 mL/100 g per minute) and is at high risk for progressing to infarction if reperfusion is not obtained. The mismatch between the Tmax > 6 seconds volume and the ischemic core volume was used to estimate the volume of salvageable tissue in DEFUSE 3 [10].

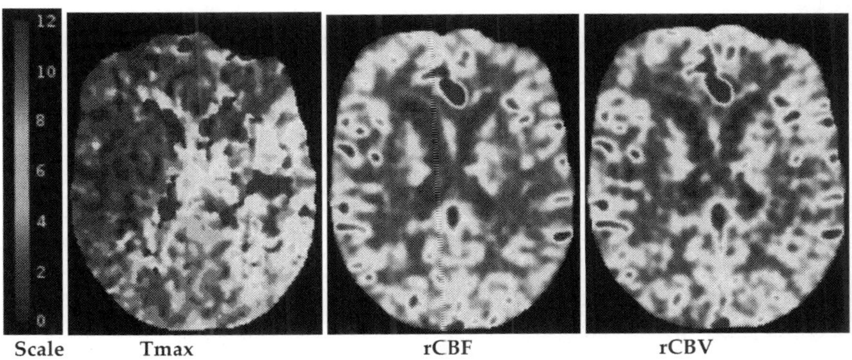

Figure 9.6. CT perfusion (CTP) scan for same patient in figure 9.4. There is normal regional Blood Volume (rBV) representing very small stroke core); prolonged Tmax > 6s in left hemisphere. This represents large mismatch (salvageable penumbra).

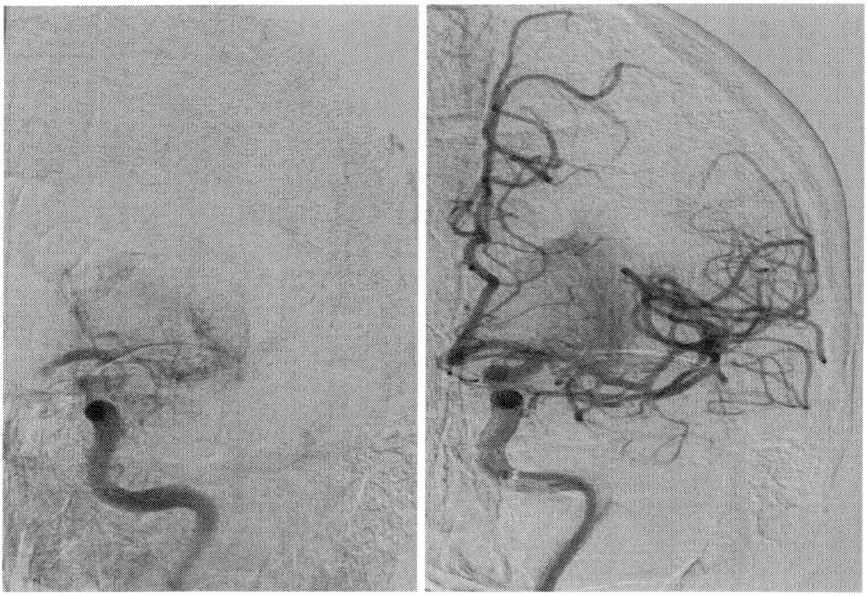

Figure 9.7. Digital subtraction angiogram (DSA) for same patient in figure 9.6. It confirms left internal carotid terminus occlusion (TICI 0) and it shows complete recanalization (TICI 3) after mechanical thrombectomy.

Table 9.1. Comparison of perfusion criteria for EVT between DEFUSE 3 and DAWN trials.

	DEFUSE 3 (10)	**DAWN** (11)
Ischemic core volume	≤ 70 mL	≤ 20 mL if age >80 ≤30 mL if age <80 and NIHSS 10–20 ≤50 mL if age <80 and NIHSS >20
Mismatch volume	≥ 15 mL and a mismatch ratio of ≥ 1.8	Not required
Vessel occlusion	M1 or ICA (cervical and intracranial)	M1 or ICA (intracranial and cervical if stent not anticipated to be required)

It is important to be aware that the Tmax maps are sensitive to delayed contrast arrival, and in some circumstances, delayed arrival does not imply critical hypoperfusion. For example, in a patient with a chronic carotid occlusion, Tmax delays may be present despite normal CBF, CBV, and mean transit times.

There are many other indications for brain CTP. It is useful in the assessment of many cerebrovascular diseases such as vasospasm after subarachnoid hemorrhage (SAH); cerebrovascular reserve by using acetazolamide challenge in patients with intracranial vascular stenosis who are potential candidates for bypass surgery or EVT; temporary balloon occlusion to assess collateral flow and cerebrovascular reserve; assessment of microvascular permeability in intracranial neoplasms; cerebral blood flow after carotid artery stent for severe stenosis; early detection of acute cerebral ischemia; follow-up study may be needed to help evaluate a patient's progress after treatment, procedure, intervention or surgery [(12) (13)].

MRI and fast MRI

Magnetic resonance image (MRI) is the most sensitive modality for acute ischemic stroke detection; however, it is more time-consuming and requires rigorous patient screening for metal objects (and cannot be done with most pacemakers). Thus, most standard acute stroke protocols do not rely on MRI as first choice.

MRI can show number of early signs of stroke that are more vivid than on NCCT (Figure 9.8). MR can also predict the time of onset based of signal changes on different sequences. Temporal evolution of strokes is typically categorized into hyperacute (0–6 h), acute (6–24 h), subacute (24 h to approximately 2 weeks), and chronic stroke (>2 weeks old) [(14)].

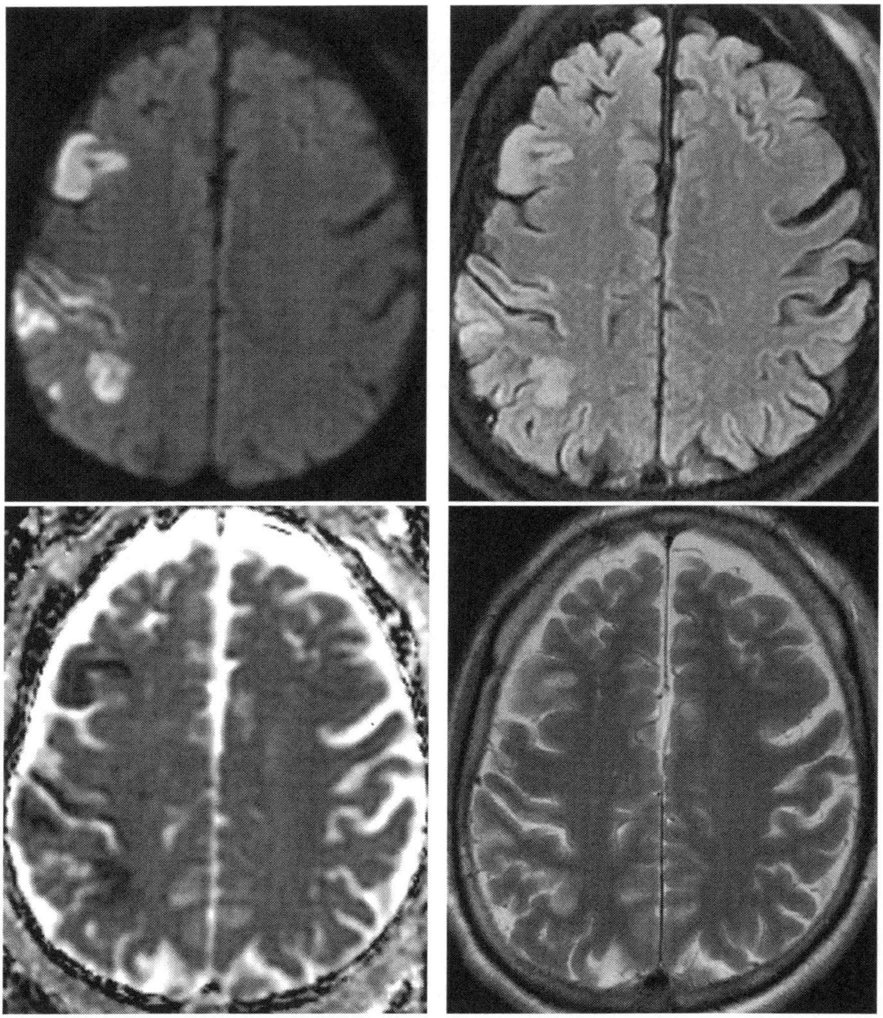

Figure 9.8
MRI images shows subacute ischemic stroke in right MCA area. DWI (upper left) show high signal; while FLAIR (upper right) shows high intensity in same areas. Echo gradient (left lower) shows dark areas that correlate with bright areas on DWI (confirming the ischemic nature of DWI changes). T2, shows brighter signal in same areas.

Diffusion-weighted Imaging (DWI)

The sensitivity of DWI is much higher than the sensitivity of most NCCT. The main sign on DWI is signal intensity change and it offers a valuable tool in acute stroke assessment due to the short time frame to detect ischemia.

FLAIR Images

Changes in fluid-attenuated inversion recovery (FLAIR) signal intensity (high intensity) start after the first 3 hours. Thus, combining data from DWI and FLAIR, providers can estimate time of onset of the suspected ischemia.

T1- and T2-weighted Images

T1 and T2 changes become visible 16 and 8 hours respectively after the onset of ischemic stroke. Thus, they have no significant value with acute stroke detection. However, in the case of a large vessel stroke, loss of flow voids (due to clot) can be detected in the large arteries on T1 and T2 (Figure 9.9).

A fast MRI protocol should ideally include DWI, FLAIR and T2 sequences. The purpose is to obtain quick (no longer than 15 minutes) images to diagnose acute stroke and assess the volume of stroke without delaying care.

▪ MR angiogram (MRA)

MRA is broadly divided into non-contrast and contrast-enhanced techniques. Non-contrast MRA can be acquired with phase contrast (PC) or time of flight (TOF) techniques, and both can be acquired as 2D slabs (for neck vessels) or 3D volumes (for cerebral vessels) [15] (Figure 9.10 and Table 9.2).

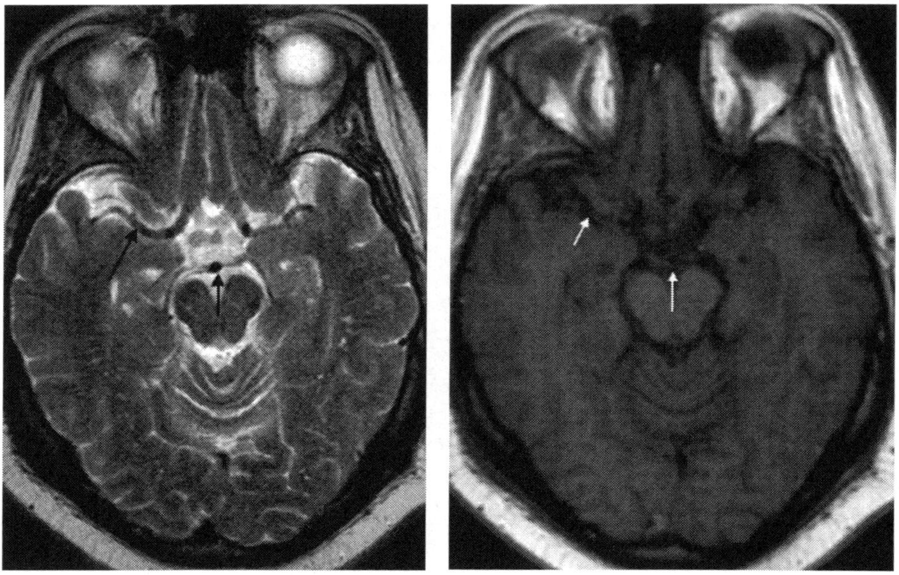

Figure 9.9. T2 (left) and T1 (right) images showing flow void (arrows) in basilar artery and right middle cerebral artery.

Table 9.2. Different types of MR angiogram (MRA).

Non-Contrast MRA (15)			
2D Time-of-Flight MRA	**3D Time-of-Flight MRA**	**Phase Contrast MRA**	**3D Phase Contrast MRA**
First MRA technique Detect inflow of blood that is fully magnetized Often used for imaging the venous system Sensitive to patient motion	"workhorse" of MRA Based on the inflow of blood into the imaging volume Provides higher signal-to-noise ratio with greater resolution	Enables the quantitative measuring of velocity	Obtains a magnitude image as well as flow image

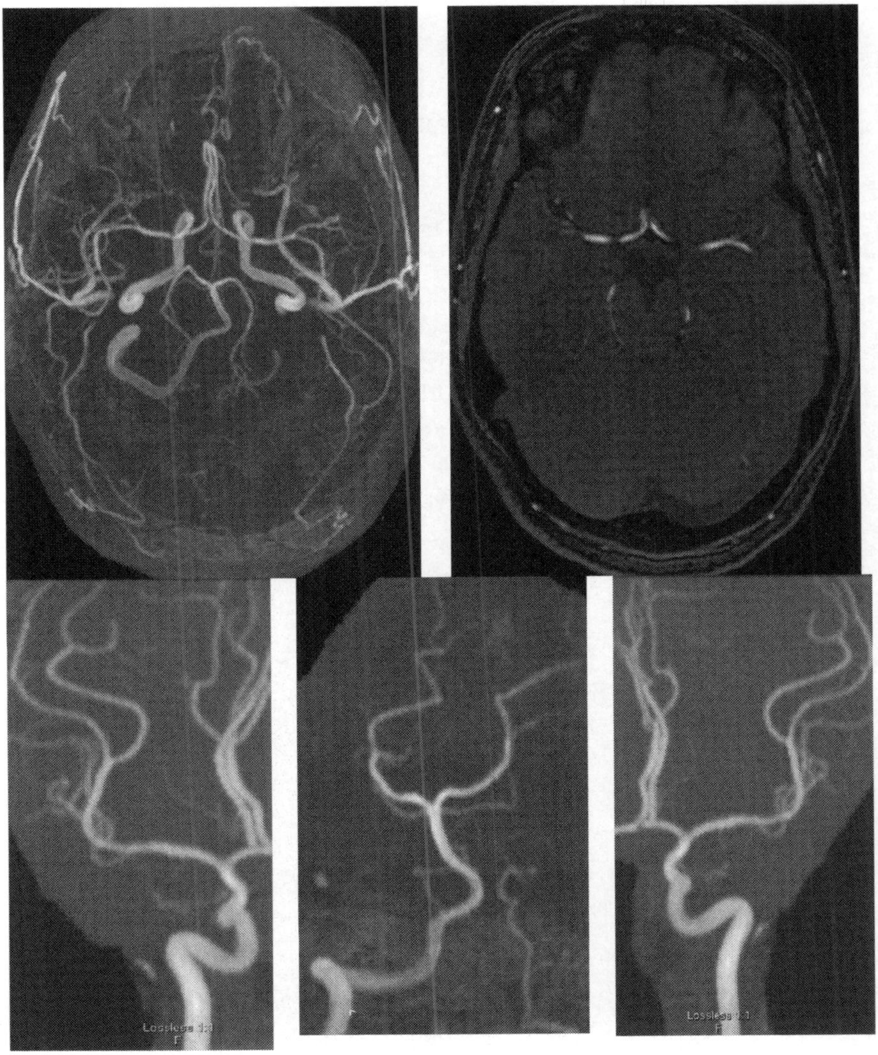

Figure 9.10. Examples of 3D Time-of-Flight (TOF) MRA. Upper left is collapse image. Upper right is source images. Lower images are 3D images of (from left to right) right MCA, basilar artery and left MCA.

MRA with contrast involves administration of IV gadolinium. The big advantage of contrast-enhanced MRA is that it is very sensitive to slow flow. A narrowly occluded artery is imaged nicely with contrast-enhanced MRA [(15)].

▪ Kidney precautions with contrast

This topic is very important to discuss because CTA and CTP are becoming standard of care for severe acute stroke work up. Treating physicians very often have to make complex decisions and may be placed under the dilemma of risking kidneys to save the brain.

Overall, there is tendency to exaggerate the risk of contrast-induced nephropathy. This, in many occasions, results in delay in CTA/P acquisition and delay in treatment and potentially worse neurological outcome. On the other hand, treating physicians should make every effort to protect the kidneys and not let the rush to do CTA/P push them to overlook basic steps to protect kidneys especially in high risk patients [(16)].

Post Contrast Acute Kidney Injury (PC-AKI) & Contrast-Induced Nephropathy (CIN)

There are no standard criteria for the diagnosis of PC-AKI or CIN. The criteria used in the past have included percent change in the baseline serum creatinine (e.g., an increase of variously 25% to 50%) and absolute elevation from baseline serum creatinine (e.g., an increase of variously 0.5 to 2.0 mg/dL). One of the most commonly used criteria has been an absolute increase of 0.5 mg/dL over a baseline serum creatinine [(16)].

Numerous studies attempted to isolate risk factors for CIN. There is consensus that the most important risk factor is pre-existing severe renal insufficiency. Multiple other risk factors have been proposed, including diabetes mellitus (DM), dehydration, cardiovascular disease, diuretic use, advanced age, multiple myeloma, hypertension (HTN), hyperuricemia, and multiple iodinated contrast medium doses in a short time interval (<24 hours), but these have not been rigorously confirmed. Two studies have shown that PC-AKI may occur after two closely spaced doses of IV iodinated contrast medium but neither study was designed to show that the risk was higher than after one or no dose of IV contrast medium [16].

There is no agreed-upon threshold of serum creatinine elevation or eGFR declination beyond which the risk of CIN is considered so great that intravascular iodinated contrast medium should never be administered.

At the current time, there is very little evidence that IV iodinated contrast material is an independent risk factor for AKI in patients with eGFR ≥30 mL/ min/1.73m. Therefore, if a threshold for CIN risk is used at all, 30 mL/ min/1.73m seems to be the one with the greatest level of evidence. It is recommended to get baseline creatinine and eGFR in certain high-risk patients [16].

Suggested list of risk factors that may warrant renal function assessment (e.g., serum creatinine, eGFR) prior to the administration of intravascular iodinated contrast medium:

- Age > 60
- History of renal disease, including:

    Dialysis

Kidney transplant
Single kidney
Renal cancer
Renal surgery

- History of HTN requiring medical therapy
- History of DM
- Metformin or metformin-containing drug combinations

The clinical course of PC -AKI (and, presumably, CIN) depends on baseline renal function, coexisting risk factors, degree of hydration, and other factors. However, the usual course consists of a transient asymptomatic elevation in serum creatinine. Serum creatinine usually begins to rise within 24 hours of intravascular iodinated contrast medium administration, peaks within 4 days, and often returns to baseline within 7 to 10 days. It is unusual for patients to develop permanent renal dysfunction.

Prevention

Prior to contrast medium administration, adequate patient assessment and communication between radiologist and referring clinician are important. Consideration of alternative imaging strategies and an individualized risk-benefit assessment are fundamental.

Volume Expansion

The major preventive action to mitigate the risk of CIN is to provide intravenous volume expansion prior to contrast medium administration. The ideal infusion rate and volume is unknown, but isotonic fluids are preferred (Lactated Ringer's or 0.9% normal saline). One possible protocol would be 0.9% saline at 100 mL/hr, beginning 6 to 12 hours before and continuing 4 to 12 hours after, but this is only practical in the inpatient setting.

Oral hydration has also been utilized, but with less demonstrated effectiveness [16].

Not all clinical studies have shown dehydration to be a major risk factor for PC-AKI. However, in the dehydrated state, renal blood flow and GFR are decreased, the effect of iodinated contrast medium on these parameters is accentuated, and there is a theoretical concern of prolonged tubular exposure to iodinated contrast medium due to low tubular flow rates. Solomon et al studied adult patients with chronic kidney disease who underwent cardiac angiography. The reported incidence of PC-AKI was decreased by periprocedural IV volume expansion or 0.9% saline, 100 mL/h, 12 hours before to 12 hours after intravascular contrast medium administration). In another study, IV volume expansion with 0.9% saline was superior to IV volume expansion with 0.45% saline in PC-AKI risk reduction [16].

Sodium Bicarbonate

Some studies and meta-analyses of patients undergoing cardiac angiography have shown intravenous volume expansion with sodium bicarbonate to be superior to 0.9% saline in reducing the risk of PC-AKI but these results have been challenged by other meta-analyses and cannot be considered definitive at this time [16].

N-acetylcysteine

The efficacy of N-acetylcysteine to reduce the incidence of CIN is controversial. Multiple studies and a number of meta-analyses have disagreed whether this agent reduces the risk of PC-AKI. There is evidence that it reduces serum creatinine in normal volunteers without changing cystatin-C (cystatin-C is reported to be a better marker of GFR than serum creatinine). This raises the possibility that N-acetylcysteine might be simply lowering serum creatinine without actually preventing renal injury. At the current time, there is insufficient evidence of its efficacy to recommend its use. N-acetylcysteine should not be considered a substitute for appropriate pre-procedural patient screening and adequate volume expansion [16].

▪ Allergic-like and physiologic reactions to contrast [16]

Tables 9.3 and 9.4 summarize reaction types and treatment.

Table 9.3. Contrast reactions.

Acute adverse reactions (AAR) (5-15%) Immediate		Delayed Adverse Events (0.5-14%) 30 minutes to a week	
Allergic like	**Physiologic**	**Non-cutaneous**	**Cutaneous**
-Mechanism is unclear -Ig E in some reactions - Histamine release	-Mechanism through direct chemotoxicity, osmotoxicity and direct binding to activators -Dose dependent		
-Allergic reaction (rash, bronchospasm, hypotension)	-Cardiac arrhythmia -Vasovagal reaction	-Nausea -Vomiting -Fever -Drowsiness -Headache -Hypotension -Cardiovascular arrest -Iodine mumps	-Urticaria -Persistent rash -Pruritis -Angioedema
-Previous history of AAR -Atopia		-Treatment with interleukin-2 - Nonionic dimeric contrast	-Treatment with interleukin-2 - Nonionic dimeric contrast
Contrast media causes exacerbation of Myasthenia Gravis.			

Table 9.4. A guide to management of contrast-induced reactions.

<table>
<tr><th colspan="2">The American College of Radiology (ACR) contrast reaction card</th></tr>
<tr>
<td>
Example premedication regimen

Methylprednisolone 32 mg PO 12, 2 hrs prior +/- Benadryl 50 mg PO 1 hr prior.
OR
Prednisone 50 mg PO 13, 7, 1 hours prior +/- Benadryl 50 mg PO 1 hr prior.
OR
Hydrocortisone 200 mg IV 5 hrs and 1 hr prior and Benadryl 50 mg IV 1 hr prior.
(urgent, NPO only, ER, inpatient)

Contrast extravasation

Elevate arm, cool compress, remove rings. Observe. Consider surgical consultation for decreased perfusion, sensation, strength, active range of motion, or increasing pain.

Hypotension with Tachycardia

1-Preserve IV access, monitor vitals q 15m.
2-O2 6-10 L/min by face mask.
3-Elevate legs > 60 degrees.
4-IVF 0.9% NS wide open.
5-Epinephrine 0.3 cc of 1:1000 IM (or auto-injector) OR Epi 1 cc of 1:10,000 IV with slow flush or IV fluids.
6-Call 911 or CODE BLUE

Hypotension with Bradycardia

1-Preserve IV access; monitor vitals2.
2-O2 6-10 L/min by face mask.
3-levate legs > 60 degrees.
4-IVF 0.9% NS wide open.
5-Atropine 0.6-1.0 mg IV if refractory
</td>
<td>
Hives/Diffuse erythema

1- Observation; monitor vitals q 15 min. Preserve IV access2.
2 -If associated with hypotension or respiratory distress then considered Anaphylaxis:

o O2 6-10 L/min by face mask
o IVF 0.9% NS wide open; elevate legs > 60°
o Epinephrine 0.3 cc of 1:1000 IM (or auto-injector) OR Epi 1 cc of 1:10,000 IV with slow flush or IV fluids
o Call 911 or CODE BLUE.

3-If ONLY skin findings but severe or progressive may consider Benadryl 50 mg PO, IM, IV but may cause or worsen hypotension

Laryngeal edema (inspiratory stridor)

1-Preserve IV access, monitor vitals.
2-O2 6-10 L/ min by face mask.
3-Epinephrine 0.3 cc of 1:1000 IM (or auto-injector) OR Epi 1 cc of 1:10,000 IV with slow flush or IV fluids.
4-Call 911 or CODE BLUE

Bronchospasm (expiratory wheezing)

1-Preserve IV access, monitor vitals.
2-O2 6-10 L/min by face mask.
3-B2 agonist inhaler 2 puffs; repeat x 3.
4-If not responding or severe, then use Epinephrine 0.3 cc of 1:1000 IM (or auto-injector) OR Epi 1 cc of 1:10,000 IV with slow flush or IV fluids.
5-Call 911 or CODE BLUE
</td>
</tr>
</table>

References

1. *Imaging Recommendations for Acute Stroke and Transient Ischemic Attack Patients: A Joint Statement by the American Society of Neuroradiology, the American College of Radiology and the Society of NeuroInterventional Surgery.* Max Wintermark, MD MAS, Pina Sanelli, MD MPH, Gregory W. Albers, MD. 11, s.l. : AJNR Am J Neuroradiol, 2013, Vol. 34.
2. *Immediate computed tomography scanning of acute stroke is cost-effective and improves quality of life.* Wardlaw JM, Seymour J, Cairns J, Keir S, Lewis S, Sandercock P. 11, s.l. : Stroke, 2004, Vol. 35.
3. *Early signs of brain infarction at CT: observer reliability and outcome after thrombolytic treatment--systematic review.* Wardlaw JM, Mielke O. 2, s.l. : Radiology, 2005, Vol. 235.
4. *Lack of clinical significance of early ischemic changes on computed tomography in acute stroke.* Patel SC, Levine SR, Tilley BC, Grotta JC,. 22, s.l. : JAMA, 2001, Vol. 286.
5. *Prevalence and significance of hyperdense middle cerebral artery in acute stroke.* Leys D, Pruvo JP, Godefroy O, Rondepierre P, Leclerc X. 3, s.l. : Stroke, 1992, Vol. 23.
6. *Use of the Alberta Stroke Program Early CT Score (ASPECTS) for Assessing CT Scans in Patients with Acute Stroke.* J. H. Warwick Pexman, Philip A. Barber, Michael D. Hill. 8, s.l. : American Journal of Neuroradiology, 2001, Vol. 22.
7. *CT angiography in the evaluation of acute stroke.* Shrier DA, Tanaka H, Numaguchi Y. 6, s.l. : AJNR Am J Neuroradiol, 1997, Vol. 18.
8. *Should CT Angiography be a Routine Component of Acute Stroke Imaging?* Vanja Douglas, MD, Michel Shamy, MD, MA, FRCPC, and Pratik Bhattacharya, MD, MPH. 3, s.l. : Neurohospitalist, 2015, Vol. 5.
9. *Cerebral Blood Flow Is the Optimal CT PerfusionParameter for Assessing Infarct Core.* Bruce C.V. Campbell, MBBS, BMedSc, FRACP, Søren Christensen, PhD and Christopher R. Levi, MBBS, FRACP. s.l. : Stroke, 2011, Vol. 42.
10. *Thrombectomy for Stroke at 6 to 16 Hours with Selection by Perfusion Imaging.* Gregory W. Albers, M.D., Michael P. Marks, M.D., Stephanie Kemp, B.S. s.l. : The New England Journal of Medicine, 2018, Vol. 378.
11. *Thrombectomy 6 to 24 Hours after Stroke with a Mismatch between Deficit and Infarct.* Raul G. Nogueira, M.D., Ashutosh P. Jadhav, M.D., Ph.D., Diogo C. Haussen, M.D. s.l. : The New England Journal of Medicine, 2018, Vol. 378.
12. *Diagnosing Vasospasm After Subarachnoid Hemorrhage: CTA and CTP.* Wilson CD, Shankar JJ. 3, s.l. : Can J Neurol Sci, 2014, Vol. 41.
13. *Cerebrovascular Reserve and Stroke Risk in Patients with Carotid Stenosis or Occlusion: A Systematic Review and Meta-Analysis.* Ajay Gupta, MD,1,* J. Levi Chazen, MD,1 Maya Hartman, MD MBA,. 11, s.l. : Stroke, 2012, Vol. 43.
14. *Sequence-specific MR Imaging Findings That Are Useful in Dating Ischemic Stroke.* Laura M. Allen, Anton N. Hasso, Jason Handwerker,. 5, s.l. : RdaioGraphics, 2012, Vol. 32.
15. González, R. [Online] NDERBILT UNIV, Sep 14, 2012. Conventional MRI and MR Angiography of Stroke.
16. Media, ACR Committee on Drugsand Contrast. *ACR Manual on Contrast Media.* [Online] 2018. https://www.acr.org/-/media/ACR/Files/Clinical-Resources/Contrast_Media.pdf.

10

Criteria for IV tPA & EVT and ASA/AHA Guidelines

This chapter focuses on guiding criteria for medical and interventional treatment for acute ischemic stroke (AIS) and on latest guidelines for early management of AIS. The author elected not to discuss details about clinical evidence of IV tPA because this is already established treatment modality and the evidence has been discussed in many other books.

This chapter elaborates on guiding principles for endovascular treatment (EVT) of AIS. It also summarizes the most recent AHA / ASA guidelines for emergent AIS treatment for completeness so this book (especially this chapter) can be used as a quick reference when treating AIS patients.

▪ Criteria for IV tPA

IV tPA is FDA approved and it is now standard of care for AIS patients who fulfill inclusion criteria and do not have any of the exclusion criteria (Table 10.1). The relative exclusion criteria are not absolute, and an experienced treating physician may proceed if benefits of IV tPA are more than risks. The following table summarizes inclusion and exclusion criteria for IV tPA.

Table 10.1. Inclusion and exclusion criteria of IV tPA.

Inclusion and exclusion criteria for administering IV tPA in acute ischemic stroke (AIS) within 4.5 hours from symptom onset [(2)(3)]
Inclusion criteria Diagnosis of ischemic stroke causing measurable neurological deficit Onset of symptoms <3 hours before treatment begins Age ≥18 y
Exclusion criteria Significant head trauma or prior stroke in the previous 3 months Symptoms suggest SAH Arterial puncture at non-compressible site in previous 7 days History of previous intracranial hemorrhage Intracranial neoplasm, AVM, or aneurysm Recent intracranial or intraspinal surgery Elevated blood pressure (systolic >185 mm Hg or diastolic >110 mm Hg) Active internal bleeding Acute bleeding diathesis, including but not limited to Platelet count <100 000/mm^3 Heparin received within 48 h resulting in abnormally elevated aPTT above the upper limit of normal Current use of anticoagulant with INR >1.7 or PT >15 seconds Current use of direct thrombin inhibitors or direct factor Xa inhibitors with elevated sensitive laboratory tests (eg, aPTT, INR, platelet count, ECT, TT, or appropriate factor Xa activity assays) Blood glucose concentration <50 mg/dL (2.7 mmol/L) CT demonstrates multilobar infarction (hypodensity >1/3 cerebral hemisphere) **Relative exclusion criteria** Recent experience suggests that under some circumstances, with careful consideration and weighting of risk to benefit, patients may receive fibrinolytic therapy despite ≥1 relative contraindication. Consider risk to benefit of IV tPA administration carefully if any of these relative

contraindications is present

- Only minor or rapidly improving stroke symptoms (clearing spontaneously)
- Pregnancy
- Seizure at onset with postictal residual neurological impairments
- Major surgery or serious trauma within previous 14 days
- Recent gastrointestinal or urinary tract hemorrhage (within previous 21 days)
- Recent acute myocardial infarction (within previous 3 months)

Notes

The checklist includes some FDA-approved indications and contraindications for administration of IV tPA for acute ischemic stroke. Recent guideline revisions have modified the original FDA-approved indications. A physician with expertise in acute stroke care may modify this list.

Onset time is defined as either the witnessed onset of symptoms or the time last known normal if symptom onset was not witnessed.

In patients without recent use of OACs or heparin, treatment with IV tPA can be initiated before availability of coagulation test results but should be discontinued if INR is >1.7 or PT is abnormally elevated by local laboratory standards.

In patients without a history of thrombocytopenia, treatment with IV tPA can be initiated before availability of platelet count but should be discontinued if platelet count is <100 000/mm3

Additional exclusion criteria for 3-4.5 hours window

- Age > 80
- History of prior stroke AND diabetes
- Any anticoagulant use prior to admission (even if INR <1.7)
- NIHSS >25
- CT findings involving more than 1/3 of the MCA territory (as evidenced by hypodensity, sulcal effacement or mass effect estimated by visual inspection or ABC/2>100 cc)

Table 10.2. Level of evidence symbols used in guidelines.

Class (Strength) of Recommendation	Level (Quality) of Evidence
Class I (Strong) Benefit >>>Risk Suggested phrases for writing recommendations: Is recommended Is indicated/useful/effective/beneficial Should be performed/administered/other Comparative-effectiveness Phrases: • Treatment/strategy A is recommended/indicated in preference to treatment B • Treatment A should be chosen over treatment B	***Level A*** • High-quality evidence from more than 1 RCT • Meta-analysis of high quality RCTs • One or more RCTs corroborated by high-quality studies
Class IIa (Moderate) Benefit >>Risk Suggested phrases for writing recommendations: Is reasonable Can be useful/effective/beneficial Comparative-effectiveness Phrases: • Treatment/strategy A is probably recommended/indicated in preference to B • It is reasonable to choose treatment A over treatment B	***Level B-R (Randomized)*** • Moderate-quality evidence from 1 or more RCTs • Meta-analyses of moderate-quality RCTs
Class IIb (Weak) Benefit ≥ Risk Suggested Phrases for writing recommendations: • May/might be reasonable • May/might be considered • Usefulness/effectiveness is unknown/unclear/uncertain or not well established	***Level B-NR (Nonrandomized)*** • Moderate-quality evidence from 1 or more well-designed, well-executed nonrandomized studies, observational studies, or registry studies • Meta-analyses of such studies
Class III: No Benefit (Moderate) Benefit= Risk Suggested phrases for writing recommendations: • Is not recommended • Is not indicated/useful/effective/beneficial • Should not be performed/administered/other	***Level C-LD (Limited Data)*** • Randomized or nonrandomized observational or registry studies with limitations of design or execution • Meta-analyses of such studies • Physiological or mechanistic studies in human subjects
Class III*: Harm (Strong) Risk > Benefit Suggested phrases for writing recommendations: • Potentially harmful • Causes harm • Associated with excess morbidity/mortality • Should not be performed/administered/other	***Level C-EO (Expert Opinion)*** • Consensus of expert opinion based on clinical experience

▪ EVT indications [2]

3% to 22% of patients with AIS are potentially eligible for mechanical thrombectomy, depending on the specific selection criteria used. Time of symptom onset (or last known well), magnitude of early ischemic change on initial imaging, clinical severity of stroke symptoms, pre-stroke level of functioning and anatomic location of the LVO are the most important determinants of candidacy for mechanical thrombectomy.

There is high-level data from multiple RCTs and registries in support of thrombectomy in appropriately selected patients, up to 24 hours from symptom onset or last known well, including wake-up strokes (Chapter 8). There is insufficient evidence to evaluate the safety and efficacy of thrombectomy >24 hours from symptom onset. Presently, only limited experience with thrombectomy of anterior circulation LVO after 24 hours has been reported.

The Society of Neurointerventional Surgery (SNIS) embraces the following recommendations:

Time from symptom onset

For anterior circulation AIS, thrombectomy is indicated in select patients up to 16 hours from symptom onset or time last known well for unwitnessed strokes, including wake-up strokes [class I, level A], and is indicated in select patients up to 24 hours from last known normal [class IIa, level B]. This replaces the 2015 SNIS guidelines in which thrombectomy recommendations were limited to the first 6 hours of symptom onset.

Imaging

In patients with anterior circulation AIS within the first 6 hours of symptom onset and *either* CT ASPECTS ≥6, MRI DWI ASPECTS ≥6, moderate-to-good collateral status on multiphase CT angiography (>50% MCA territory), small (<50–70mL) core infarct volumes, and / or significant penumbral to core mismatch on advanced perfusion imaging (CTP or MRI-DWI-PWI), thrombectomy is indicated [class I, level A].

Thrombectomy may be reasonable within the first 6 hours of symptom onset in patients with a large core infarct volume such as CT ASPECTS of <6, MRI DWI or CTP-estimated core volume >70 mL [class IIa, level A].

In patients with anterior circulation AIS due to intracranial ICA and / or M1 occlusion within 6–24 hours of symptom onset who meet the advanced MRI DWI-PWI or CTP imaging criteria for DAWN or DEFUSE 3, thrombectomy is indicated [class I, level B].

Thrombectomy may be indicated in carefully selected patients with anterior circulation AIS within 6–24 hours of symptom onset who do not meet imaging criteria for DAWN and DEFUSE 3 but otherwise have a 'favorable' imaging profile such as CT ASPECTS of 6–10, MRI DWI ASPECTS of 6–10, moderate-to-good collateral status on mCTA, or small (<70 mL) core infarct on advanced MRI DWI-PWI or CTP imaging [class IIb, level B-NR (non-randomized)].

Location of LVO

Thrombectomy is indicated in patients with occlusions of the ICA (including intracranial, cervical segments or tandem occlusion) and M1 / M2 MCA [class I, level A]. This replaces the

2015 SNIS guidelines in which thrombectomy recommendations were limited to ICA and MCA M1 LVO locations.

The benefit of thrombectomy in more distal segments, such as MCA M3 or anterior cerebral artery is unclear. Thrombectomy of such patients may be reasonable in some cases and should be considered on a case-by-case basis [class IIb, level B-NR].

Stroke severity

Thrombectomy is indicated in patients with anterior circulation LVO with NIHSS score ≥6 [class I, level A].

Thrombectomy may be considered in patients with anterior circulation AIS and NIHSS score <6 when associated with disabling symptoms [class IIa, level B-NR]. However, care should be taken when treating these patients to keep complication and hemorrhagic rates below those reported in RCTs.

Age and baseline level of functioning

Age >80 years should not be used as a contraindication for thrombectomy [class IIa, level A].

The benefit of thrombectomy in patients with baseline mRS score >1 is unknown.

▪ AHA/ASA acute stroke guidelines (3)

Table 10.3. AHA / ASA emergent stroke treatment 2018 guidelines.

1. Prehospital Stroke Management and Systems of Care	
Prehospital Systems	
All stroke stakeholders should design and implement protocols focused on stroke systems and the need to seek emergency care (by calling 9-1-1) in a rapid manner. These programs should be sustained over time and designed to reach racially / ethnically, age, and sex diverse populations.	I BR
Activation of the 9-1-1 system by patients or other members of the public is strongly recommended. 9-1-1 dispatchers should make stroke a priority dispatch, and transport times should be minimized.	I BNR
To increase both the number of patients who are treated and the quality of care, educational stroke programs for physicians, hospital personnel, and EMS personnel are recommended.	I BNR
EMS Assessment and Management	
The use of a stroke assessment system by first aid providers, including EMS dispatch personnel, is recommended.	I BNR
EMS personnel should begin the initial management of stroke in the field. Implementation of a stroke protocol to be used by EMS personnel is strongly encouraged.	I BNR
EMS personnel should provide prehospital notification to the receiving hospital that a suspected stroke patient is en-route so that the appropriate hospital resources may be mobilized before patient arrival.	I BNR
EMS Systems	
EMS leaders, in coordination with local, regional, and state agencies and in consultation with medical authorities and local experts, should develop triage paradigms and protocols to ensure that patients with a known or suspected stroke are rapidly identified and assessed by use of a validated and standardized instrument for stroke screening, such as the FAST (face, arm, speech test) scale, Los Angeles Prehospital Stroke Screen, or Cincinnati Prehospital Stroke Scale.	I BNR
Regional systems of stroke care should be developed. These should consist of the following: (a) Healthcare facilities that provide initial emergency care, including administration of IV tPA, and, (b) Centers capable of performing endovascular stroke treatment with comprehensive periprocedural care to which rapid transport can be arranged when appropriate.	I A
Patients with a positive stroke screen and / or a strong suspicion of stroke	I

should be transported rapidly to the closest healthcare facilities that can capably administer IV tPA.	BNR
When several IV tPA–capable hospital options exist within a defined geographic region, the benefit of bypassing the closest to bring the patient to one that offers a higher level of stroke care, including mechanical thrombectomy, is uncertain. Further research is needed. At least 6 stroke severity scales targeted at recognition of large vessel occlusion (LVO) in the prehospital setting to facilitate transfer to endovascular centers have been published. All the scales were initially derived from data sets of confirmed stroke cases or selected prehospital cases, and there has been only limited study of their performance in the prehospital setting. For prehospital patients with suspected LVO by a stroke severity scale, the Mission: Lifeline Severity–based Stroke Triage Algorithm for EMS recommends direct transport to a comprehensive stroke center if the travel time to the comprehensive stroke center is <15 additional minutes compared with the travel time to the closest primary stroke center or acute stroke-ready hospital. However, at this time, there is insufficient evidence to recommend 1 scale over the other or a specific threshold of additional travel time for which bypass of a primary stroke center or acute stroke-ready hospital is justifiable. Given the known impact of delays to IV tPA on outcomes, the known impact of delays to mechanical thrombectomy on outcome, and the anticipated delays in transport for mechanical thrombectomy in eligible patients originally triaged to a non-endovascular center, the Mission: Lifeline algorithm may be a reasonable guideline in some circumstances. Customization of the guideline to optimize patient outcomes will be needed to account for local and regional factors, including the availability of endovascular centers, door in–door out times for non-endovascular stroke centers, interhospital transport times, and DTN and door-to-puncture times. Rapid, protected, collaborative, regional quality review, including EMS agencies and hospitals, is recommended for operationalized bypass algorithms	IIb BNR
Hospital Stroke Capabilities	
Certification of stroke centers by an independent external body, such as Center for Improvement in Healthcare Quality, Det Norske Veritas, Healthcare Facilities Accreditation Program, and The Joint Commission (TJC),* or a state health department, is recommended. Additional medical centers should seek such certification. *AHA has a cobranded, revenue-generating stroke certification with TJC.	I BNR
Hospital Stroke Teams	
An organized protocol for the emergency evaluation of patients with suspected stroke is recommended.	I BNR
It is recommended that door to needle (DTN) time goals be established. A primary goal of achieving DTN times within 60 minutes in ≥ 50% of AIS patients treated with IV tPA should be established	I BNR
It may be reasonable to establish a secondary DTN time goal of achieving DTN times within 45 minutes in ≥50% of patients with AIS who were treated with IV tPA.	IIb CEO
Designation of an acute stroke team that includes physicians, nurses, and laboratory/radiology personnel is recommended. Patients with stroke should have a careful clinical assessment, including neurological examination.	I BNR
Multicomponent quality improvement initiatives, which include ED education and multidisciplinary teams with access to neurological	I A

expertise, are recommended to safely increase IV thrombolytic treatment.	
Telemedicine	
For sites without in-house imaging interpretation expertise, teleradiology systems approved by the US Food and Drug Administration are recommended for timely review of brain imaging in patients with suspected acute stroke.	I A
When implemented within a telestroke network, teleradiology systems approved by the US Food and Drug Administration are useful in supporting rapid imaging interpretation in time for IV tPA administration decision making.	I A
Because of the limited distribution and availability of neurological, neurosurgical, and radiological expertise, the use of telemedicine/telestroke resources and systems can be beneficial and should be supported by healthcare institutions, governments, payers, and vendors as one method to ensure adequate 24/7 coverage and care of acute stroke patients in a variety of settings.	IIa CEO
Telestroke/teleradiology evaluations of AIS patients can be effective for correct IV tPA eligibility decision making.	IIa BR
Administration of IV tPA guided by telestroke consultation for patients with AIS may be as safe and as beneficial as that of stroke centers.	IIb BNR
Providing tPA decision-making support via telephone consultation to community physicians is feasible and safe and may be considered when a hospital has access to neither an in person stroke team nor a telestroke system.	IIb C LD
Organization and Integration of Components	
It may be useful for primary stroke centers and other healthcare facilities that provide initial emergency care, including administration of IV tPA, to develop the capability of performing emergency noninvasive intracranial vascular imaging to most appropriately select patients for transfer for endovascular intervention and to reduce the time to EVT	IIb CLD
Mechanical thrombectomy requires the patient to be at an experienced stroke center with rapid access to cerebral angiography, qualified neurointerventionalists, and a comprehensive periprocedural care team. Systems should be designed, executed, and monitored to emphasize expeditious assessment and treatment. Outcomes for all patients should be tracked. Facilities are encouraged to define criteria that can be used to credential individuals who can perform safe and timely intra-arterial revascularization procedures	I CEO
All hospitals caring for stroke patients within a stroke system of care should develop, adopt, and adhere to care protocols that reflect current care guidelines as established by national and international professional	I CEO

organizations and state and federal agencies and laws	
Different services within a hospital that may be transferring patients through a continuum of care, as well as different hospitals that may be transferring patients to other facilities, should establish hand-off and transfer protocols and procedures that ensure safe and efficient patient care within and between facilities. Protocols for interhospital transfer of patients should be established and approved beforehand so that efficient patient transfers can be accomplished at all hours of the day and night	I CEO
It may be beneficial for government agencies and third-party payers to develop and implement reimbursement schedules for patients with acute stroke that reflect the demanding care and expertise that such patients require to achieve an optimal outcome, regardless of whether they receive a specific medication or procedure.	IIb CEO
Establishment of Data Repositories	
Participation in a stroke data repository is recommended to promote consistent adherence to current treatment guidelines, to allow continuous quality improvement, and to improve patient outcomes	I BNR
Healthcare institutions should organize a multidisciplinary quality improvement committee to review and monitor stroke care quality benchmarks, indicators, evidence-based practices, and outcomes. The formation of a clinical process improvement team and the establishment of a stroke care data bank are helpful for such quality of care assurances. The data repository can be used to identify the gaps or disparities in quality stroke care. Once the gaps have been identified, specific interventions can be initiated to address these gaps or disparities.	I BNR
Continuous quality improvement processes, implemented by each major element of a stroke system of care and the system as a whole, can be useful in improving patient care or outcomes.	IIa BNR
Stroke outcome measures should include adjustments for baseline severity.	I BNR
2. Emergency Evaluation and Treatment	
Stroke Scale	
The use of a stroke severity rating scale, preferably the NIHSS, is recommended.	I BNR
Brain Imaging	
All patients admitted to hospital with suspected acute stroke should receive brain imaging evaluation on arrival to hospital. In most cases, non-contrast CT (NCCT) will provide the necessary information to make decisions about acute management.	I BNR
Systems should be established so that brain imaging studies can be	I

performed within 20 minutes of arrival in the ED in at least 50% of patients who may be candidates for IV tPA and/or mechanical thrombectomy.	BNR
There remains insufficient evidence to identify a threshold of acute CT hypoattenuation severity or extent that affects treatment response to IV tPA. The extent and severity of acute hypoattenuation or early ischemic changes should not be used as a criterion to withhold therapy for such patients who otherwise qualify	III BR
The CT hyperdense MCA sign should not be used as a criterion to withhold IV tPA from patients who otherwise qualify	III BR
Routine use of magnetic resonance imaging (MRI) to exclude cerebral microbleeds (CMBs) before administration of IV tPA is not recommended.	III BR
Use of imaging criteria to select ischemic stroke patients who a woke with stroke or have unclear time of symptom onset for treatment with IV tPA is not recommended outside a clinical trial	III BNR
Multimodal CT and MRI, including perfusion imaging, should not delay administration of IV tPA	III* BNR
For patients who otherwise meet criteria for EVT, a noninvasive intracranial vascular study is recommended during the initial imaging evaluation of the acute stroke patient, but should not delay IV tPA if indicated. For patients who qualify for IV tPA according to guidelines from professional medical societies, initiating IV tPA before noninvasive vascular imaging is recommended for patients who have not had noninvasive vascular imaging as part of their initial imaging assessment for stroke. Noninvasive intracranial vascular imaging should then be obtained as quickly as possible	I A
For patients who otherwise meet criteria for EVT, it is reasonable to proceed with CTA if indicated in patients with suspected intracranial LVO before obtaining a serum creatinine concentration in patients without a history of renal impairment.	IIa RNR
In patients who are potential candidates for mechanical thrombectomy, imaging of the extracranial carotid and vertebral arteries, in addition to the intracranial circulation, is reasonable to provide useful information on patient eligibility and endovascular procedural planning	IIa CEO
Additional imaging beyond CT and CTA or MRI and magnetic resonance angiography (MRA) such as perfusion studies for selecting patients for mechanical thrombectomy in <6 hours is not recommended.	III BR

Recommendation	Class / Level
In selected patients with AIS within 6 to 24 hours of last known normal who have LVO in the anterior circulation, obtaining CTP, DW-MRI, or MRI perfusion is recommended to aid in patient selection for mechanical thrombectomy, but only when imaging and other eligibility criteria from RCTs showing benefit are being strictly applied in selecting patients for mechanical thrombectomy	I A
It may be reasonable to incorporate collateral flow status into clinical decision making in some candidates to determine eligibility for mechanical thrombectomy.	IIb CLD
Other Diagnostic Tests	
Only the assessment of blood glucose must precede the initiation of IV tPA in all patients.	I BR
Baseline ECG assessment is recommended in patients presenting with AIS, but should not delay initiation of IV tPA.	I BNR
Baseline troponin assessment is recommended in patients presenting with AIS, but should not delay initiation of IV tPA.	I BNR
Usefulness of chest radiographs in the hyperacute stroke setting in the absence of evidence of acute pulmonary, cardiac, or pulmonary vascular disease is unclear. If obtained, they should not unnecessarily delay administration of IV tPA.	IIb BNR
3. General Supportive Care and Emergency Treatment	
Airway, Breathing, and Oxygenation	
Airway support and ventilatory assistance are recommended for the treatment of patients with acute stroke who have decreased consciousness or who have bulbar dysfunction that causes compromise of the airway	I CEO
Supplemental oxygen should be provided to maintain oxygen saturation >94%.	I CLD
Supplemental oxygen is not recommended in nonhypoxic patients with AIS.	III CLD
Hyperbaric oxygen (HBO) is not recommended for patients with AIS except when caused by air embolization	III BNR
Blood Pressure	
Hypotension and hypovolemia should be corrected to maintain systemic perfusion levels necessary to support organ function	I CEO
Patients who have elevated BP and are otherwise eligible for treatment with IV tPA should have their BP carefully lowered so that their systolic BP is <185 mm Hg and their diastolic BP is <110 mm Hg before IV fibrinolytic therapy is initiated.	I BNR

Until additional data become available, in patients for whom intra-arterial therapy is planned and who have not received IV thrombolytic therapy, it is reasonable to maintain BP ≤185/110 mm Hg before the procedure.	IIb BR
The usefulness of drug-induced hypertension in patients with AIS is not well established.	IIb CLD

Options to Treat Arterial Hypertension in Patients With AIS Who Are Candidates for Acute Reperfusion Therapy (Class IIb, LOE C-EO)
Patient otherwise eligible for acute reperfusion therapy except that BP is >185/110 mm Hg:
• Labetalol 10–20 mg IV over 1–2 min, may repeat 1 time; or • Nicardipine 5 mg/h IV, titrate up by 2.5 mg/h every 5–15 min, maximum 15 mg/h; whendesired BP reached, adjust to maintain proper BP limits; or • Clevidipine 1–2 mg/h IV, titrate by doubling the dose every 2–5 min until desired BP reached; maximum 21 mg/h • Other agents (eg, hydralazine, enalaprilat) may also be considered If BP is not maintained ≤185/110 mmHg, do not administer tPA
Management of BP during and after tPA or other acute reperfusion therapy to maintain BP ≤ 180/105 mm Hg:
• Monitor BP every 15 min for 2 h from the start of tPA therapy, then every 30 min for 6 h, and then every hour for 16 h
If systolic BP >180–230 mm Hg or diastolic BP >105–120 mm Hg:
• Labetalol 10 mg IV followed by continuous IV infusion 2–8 mg/min; or • Nicardipine 5 mg/h IV, titrate up to desired effect by 2.5 mg/h every 5–15 min, maximum 15 mg/h; or • Clevidipine 1–2 mg/h IV, titrate by doubling the dose every 2-5 min until desired BP reached; maximum 21 mg/h If BP not controlled or diastolic BP >140 mm Hg, consider IV sodium nitroprusside

Temperature	
Sources of hyperthermia (temperature >38°C) should be identified and treated, and antipyretic medications should be administered to lower temperature in hyperthermic patients with stroke	I CEO
The benefit of induced hypothermia for treating patients with ischemic stroke is not well established. Hypothermia should be offered only in the context of ongoing clinical trials	IIb BR
Blood Glucose	
Evidence indicates that persistent in-hospital hyperglycemia during the first 24 hours after AIS is associated with worse outcomes than normoglycemia and thus, it is reasonable to treat hyperglycemia to achieve blood glucose levels in a range of 140 to 180 mg/dL and to closely monitor	IIb CLD

to prevent hypoglycemia in patients with AIS.	
Hypoglycemia (blood glucose <60 mg/dL) should be treated in patients with AIS.	I CLD
IV tPA	
IV tPA (0.9 mg/kg, maximum dose 90 mg over 60 minutes with initial 10% of dose given as bolus over 1 minute) is recommended for selected patients who may be treated within 3 hours of ischemic stroke symptom onset or patient last known well or at baseline state. Physicians should review the criteria outlined in Table 6 to determine patient eligibility	I A
IV tPA (0.9 mg/kg, maximum dose 90 mg over 60 minutes with initial 10% of dose given as bolus over 1 minute) is also recommended for selected patients who can be treated within 3 and 4.5 hours of ischemic stroke symptom onset or patient last known well. Physicians should review the criteria outlined in Table 6 determine patient eligibility.	I BR
For otherwise eligible patients with mild stroke presenting in the 3- to 4.5-hour window, treatment with IV tPA may be reasonable. Treatment risks should be weighed against possible benefits	IIb BNR
In otherwise eligible patients who have had a previously demonstrated small number (1–10) of CMBs on MRI, administration of IV tPA is reasonable.	IIa BNR
In otherwise eligible patients who have had a previously demonstrated high burden of CMBs (>10) on MRI, treatment with IV tPA may be associated with an increased risk of sICH, and the benefits of treatment are uncertain. Treatment may be reasonable if there is the potential for substantial benefit	IIb BNR
IV tPA for adults presenting with an AIS with known sickle cell disease can be beneficial.	IIa BNR
Abciximab should not be administered concurrently with IV tPA.	III* BR
IV tPA should not be administered to patients who have received a treatment dose of low-molecular-weight heparin (LMWH) within the previous 24 hours.	III* BNR
The potential risks should be discussed during thrombolysis eligibility deliberation and weighed against the anticipated benefits during decision making.	I CEO
Given the extremely low risk of unsuspected abnormal platelet counts or coagulation studies in a population, it is reasonable that urgent IV tPA treatment not be delayed while waiting for hematologic or coagulation testing if there is no reason to suspect an abnormal test.	IIa BNR
Treating clinicians should be aware that hypoglycemia and hyperglycemia	III

may mimic acute stroke presentations and determine blood glucose levels before IV tPA initiation. IV tPA is not indicated for nonvascular conditions.	BNR
Because time from onset of symptoms to treatment has such a powerful impact on outcomes, treatment with IV tPA should not be delayed to monitor for further improvement	III* CEO
In patients undergoing fibrinolytic therapy, physicians should be prepared to treat potential emergent adverse effects, including bleeding complications and angioedema that may cause partial airway obstruction	I BNR
BP should be maintained <180/105 mm Hg for at least the first 24 hours after IV tPA treatment.	I BNR
The risk of antithrombotic therapy within the first 24 hours after treatment with IV tPA (with or without EVT) is uncertain. Use might be considered in the presence of concomitant conditions for which such treatment given in the absence of IV tPA is known to provide substantial benefit or withholding such treatment is known to cause substantial risk	IIb BNR
In patients eligible for IV tPA, benefit of therapy is time dependent, and treatment should be initiated as quickly as possible.	I A
Other IV Thrombolytics and Sonothrombolysis	
The benefit of IV defibrinogenating agents and of IV fibrinolytic agents other than tPA and tenecteplase is unproven; therefore, their administration is not recommended outside a clinical trial.	III BR
Tenecteplase administered as a 0.4-mg/kg single IV bolus has not been proven to be superior or noninferior to tPA but might be considered as an alternative to tPA in patients with minor neurological impairment and no major intracranial occlusion.	IIb BR
The use of sonothrombolysis as adjuvant therapy with IV thrombolysis is not recommended.	III BR
Mechanical Thrombectomy	
Patients eligible for IV tPA should receive IV tPA even if EVTs are being considered.	I A
In patients under consideration for mechanical thrombectomy, observation after IV tPA to assess for clinical response should not be performed	III* BR
Patients should receive mechanical thrombectomy with a stent retriever if they meet all the following criteria: (1) prestroke mRS score of 0 to 1; (2) causative occlusion of the internal carotid artery or MCA segment 1 (M1); (3) age ≥18 years; (4) NIHSS score of ≥ 6; (5) ASPECTS of ≥ 6; and (6) treatment can be initiated (groin puncture) within 6 hours of symptom onset.	I A
Although the benefits are uncertain, the use of mechanical thrombectomy	IIb

with stent retrievers may be reasonable for carefully selected patients with AIS in whom treatment can be initiated (groin puncture) within 6 hours of symptom onset and who have causative occlusion of the MCA segment 2 (M2) or MCA segment 3 (M3) portion of the MCAs	BR
Although the benefits are uncertain, the use of mechanical thrombectomy with stent retrievers may be reasonable for carefully selected patients with AIS in whom treatment can be initiated (groin puncture) within 6 hours of symptom onset and who have causative occlusion of the anterior cerebral arteries, vertebral arteries, basilar artery, or posterior cerebral arteries.	CEO
Although its benefits are uncertain,the use of mechanical thrombectomy with stent retrievers may be reasonable for patients with AIS in whom treatment can be initiated (groin puncture) within 6 hours of symptom onset and who have prestroke mRS score >1, ASPECTS <6, or NIHSS score <6, and causative occlusion of the internal carotid artery (ICA) or proximal MCA (M1). Additional randomized trial data are needed	IIb BR
In selected patients with AIS within 6 to 16 hours of last known normal who have LVO in the anterior circulation and meet other DAWN or DEFUSE 3 eligibility criteria, mechanical thrombectomy is recommended.	I A
In selected patients with AIS within 6 to 24 hours of last known normal who have LVO in the anterior circulation and meet other DAWN eligibility criteria, mechanical thrombectomy is reasonable.	IIb BR
The technical goal of the thrombectomy procedure should be reperfusion to a modified Thrombolysis in Cerebral Infarction (mTICI) 2b/3 angiographic result to maximize the probability of a good functional clinical outcome.	I A
As with IV tPA, reduced time from symptom onset to reperfusion with endovascular therapies is highly associated with better clinical outcomes. To ensure benefit, reperfusion to TICI grade 2b/3 should be achieved as early as possible within the therapeutic window.	I BR
Use of stent retrievers is indicated in preference to the Mechanical Embolus Removal in Cerebral Ischemia (MERCI) device.	I A
The use of mechanical thrombectomy devices other than stent retrievers as first-line devices for mechanical thrombectomy may be reasonable in some circumstances, but stent retrievers remain the first choice.	IIb BR
The use of a proximal balloon guide catheter or a large-bore distal-access catheter, rather than a cervical guide catheter alone, in conjunction with stent retrievers may be beneficial. Future studies should examine which systems provide the highest recanalization rates with the lowest risk for nontarget embolization	IIa CLD
Use of salvage technical adjuncts including intra-arterial thrombolysis may be reasonable to achieve mTICI 2b/3 angiographic results.	IIb CLD

EVT of tandem occlusions (both extracranial and intracranial occlusions) at the time of thrombectomy may be reasonable.	IIb BR
It is reasonable to select an anesthetic technique during endovascular therapy for AIS on the basis of individualized assessment of patient risk factors, technical performance of the procedure, and other clinical characteristics. Further randomized trial data are needed.	IIa BR
In patients who undergo mechanical thrombectomy, it is reasonable to maintain the BP ≤ 180/105 mm Hg during and for 24 hours after the procedure	IIa BNR
In patients who undergo mechanical thrombectomy with successful reperfusion, it might be reasonable to maintain BP at a level <180/105 mm Hg	IIb BNR
Other EVTs	
Initial treatment with intra-arterial thrombolysis is beneficial for carefully selected patients with major ischemic strokes of <6 hours' duration caused by occlusions of the MCA.	I BR
Regarding the previous recommendation about intra-arterial thrombolysis, these data are derived from clinical trials that no longer reflect current practice, including the use of fibrinolytic drugs that are not available. A clinically beneficial dose of intra-arterial tPA is not established, and tPA does not have US Food and Drug Administration approval for intra-arterial use. As a consequence, mechanical thrombectomy with stent retrievers is recommended over intra-arterial thrombolysis as first-line therapy	I CEO
Intra-arterial thrombolysis initiated within 6 hours of stroke onset in carefully selected patients who have contraindications to the use of IV tPA might be considered, but the consequences are unknown.	IIb CEO
Antiplatelet Treatment	
Administration of aspirin is recommended in patients with AIS within 24 to 48 hours after onset. For those treated with IV tPA, aspirin administration is generally delayed until 24 hours later but might be considered in the presence of concomitant conditions for which such treatment given in the absence of IV tPA is known to provide substantial benefit or withholding such treatment is known to cause substantial risk.	I A
Aspirin is not recommended as a substitute for acute stroke treatment in patients who are otherwise eligible for IV tPA or mechanical thrombectomy.	III BR
The efficacy of IV tirofiban and eptifibatide is not well established. Further clinical trials are needed.	IIb BR
The administration of other glycoprotein IIb/IIIa receptor antagonists,	III*

including abciximab, in the treatment of AIS is potentially harmful and should not be performed. Further research testing the safety and efficacy of these medications in patients with AIS is required	BR
In patients presenting with minor stroke, treatment for 21 days with dual antiplatelet therapy (aspirin and clopidogrel) begun within 24 hours can be beneficial for early secondary stroke prevention for a period of up to 90 days from symptom onset	IIa BR
Ticagrelor is not recommended (over aspirin) in the acute treatment of patients with minor stroke	III BR
Anticoagulants	
Urgent anticoagulation, with the goal of preventing early recurrent stroke, halting neurological worsening, or improving outcomes after AIS, is not recommended for treatment of patients with AIS.	III A
The usefulness of urgent anticoagulation in patients with severe stenosis of an internal carotid artery ipsilateral to an ischemic stroke is not well established.	IIb BNR
The safety and usefulness of short-term anticoagulation for nonocclusive, extracranial intraluminal thrombus in the setting of AIS are not well established.	IIb CLD
At present, the usefulness of argatroban, dabigatran, or other thrombin inhibitors for the treatment of patients with AIS is not well established. Further clinical trials are needed.	IIb BR
The safety and usefulness of factor Xa inhibitors in the treatment of AIS are not well established. Further clinical trials are needed.	IIb CLD
Volume Expansion/Hemodilution, Vasodilators, and Hemodynamic Augmentation	
Hemodilution by volume expansion is not recommended for treatment of patients with AIS.	III A
The administration of high-dose albumin is not recommended for the treatment of patients with AIS.	III A
The administration of vasodilatory agents, such as pentoxifylline, is not recommended for treatment of patients with AIS.	III A
At present, use of devices to augment cerebral blood flow for the treatment of patients with AIS is not well established. These devices should be used only in the setting of clinical trials	IIb BR
Neuroprotective Agents	
At present, no pharmacological or non-pharmacological treatments with putative neuroprotective actions have demonstrated efficacy in improving	III A

outcomes after ischemic stroke, and therefore, other neuroprotective agents are not recommended.	
Emergency CEA/Carotid Angioplasty & Stenting Without Intracranial Clot	
The usefulness of emergent or urgent CEA when clinical indicators or brain imaging suggests a small infarct core with large territory at risk (eg, penumbra), compromised by inadequate flow from a critical carotid stenosis or occlusion, or in the case of acute neurological deficit after CEA, in which acute thrombosis of the surgical site is suspected, is not well established.	IIb BNR
In patients with unstable neurological status (eg, stroke-in-evolution), the efficacy of emergency or urgent CEA is not well established	IIb BNR
Transcranial near-infrared laser therapy is not recommended for the treatment of AIS	III BR
4. In-Hospital Management of AIS: General Supportive Care	
Stroke Units	
The use of comprehensive specialized stroke care (stroke units) that incorporates rehabilitation is recommended.	I A
The use of standardized stroke care order sets is recommended to improve general management.	I BNR
Supplemental Oxygen	
Airway support and ventilatory assistance are recommended for the treatment of patients with acute stroke who have decreased consciousness or who have bulbar dysfunction that causes compromise of the airway	I CEO
Supplemental oxygen should be provided to maintain oxygen saturation >94%.	I CLD
Supplemental oxygen is not recommended in nonhypoxic patients hospitalized with AIS	III BR
Blood Pressure	
In patients with AIS, early treatment of hypertension is indicated when required by comorbid conditions (eg, concomitant acute coronary event, acute heart failure, aortic dissection, postthrombolysis sICH, or preeclampsia/eclampsia). Lowering BP initially by 15% is probably safe	I CEO
In patients with BP <220/120 mm Hg who did not receive IV tPA or EVT and do not have a comorbid condition requiring acute antihypertensive treatment, initiating or reinitiating treatment of hypertension within the first 48 to 72 hours after an AIS is not effective to prevent death or dependency	III A

In patients with BP ≥ 220/120 mm Hg who did not receive IV tPA or EVT and have no comorbid conditions requiring acute antihypertensive treatment, the benefit of initiating or reinitiating treatment of hypertension within the first 48 to 72 hours is uncertain. It might be reasonable to lower BP by 15% during the first 24 hours after onset of stroke.	IIb CEO
Although no solid data are available to guide selection of medications for BP lowering after AIS, the antihypertensive medications and doses included in Table 5 are reasonable options.	IIa CEO
Starting or restarting antihypertensive therapy during hospitalization in patients with BP >140/90 mm Hg who are neurologically stable is safe and is reasonable to improve long-term BP control unless contraindicated.	IIa BR
Hypotension and hypovolemia should be corrected to maintain systemic perfusion levels necessary to support organ function.	I CEO
Temperature	
Sources of hyperthermia (temperature >38°C) should be identified and treated. Antipyretic medications should be administered to lower temperature in hyperthermic patients with stroke	I CEO
The benefit of induced hypothermia for treating patients with ischemic stroke is not well established. Hypothermia should be offered only in the context of ongoing clinical trials.	IIb BR
Glucose	
Evidence indicates that persistent in-hospital hyperglycemia during the first 24 hours after AIS is associated with worse outcomes than normoglycemia, and thus, it is reasonable to treat hyperglycemia to achieve blood glucose levels in a range of 140 to 180 mg/dL and to closely monitor to prevent hypoglycemia	IIa CLD
Hypoglycemia (blood glucose <60 mg/dL) should be treated in patients with AIS	I CLD
Dysphagia Screening	
Dysphagia screening before the patient begins eating, drinking, or receiving oral medications is reasonable to identify patients at increased risk for aspiration.	IIa CLD
It is reasonable for dysphagia screening to be performed by a speech-language pathologist or other trained healthcare provider.	IIa CLD
An instrumental evaluation is reasonable for those patients suspected of aspiration to verify the presence/absence of aspiration and to determine the physiological reasons for the dysphagia to guide the treatment plan.	IIb BNR
It is not well-established which instrument to choose for evaluation of	I

swallowing with sensory testing, but the choice may be based on instrument availability or other considerations (ie, fiberoptic endoscopic evaluation of swallowing, videofluoroscopy, fiberoptic endoscopic evaluation).	CLD
Nutrition	
Enteral diet should be started within 7 days of admission after an acute stroke.	I BR
For patients with dysphagia, it is reasonable to initially use nasogastric tubes for feeding in the early phase of stroke (starting within the first 7 days) and to place percutaneous gastrostomy tubes in patients with longer anticipated persistent inability to swallow safely (>2–3 weeks).	IIa CEO
Nutritional supplements are reasonable to consider for patients who are malnourished or at risk of malnourishment.	IIb BR
Implementing oral hygiene protocols to reduce the risk of pneumonia after stroke may be reasonable	I BNR
Deep Vein Thrombosis Prophylaxis	
In immobile stroke patients without contraindications, intermittent pneumatic compression (IPC) in addition to routine care (aspirin and hydration) is recommended over routine care to reduce the risk of deep vein thrombosis (DVT).	I BR
The benefit of prophylactic-dose subcutaneous heparin (unfractionated heparin [UFH] or LMWH) in immobile patients with AIS is not well established.	IIb A
When prophylactic anticoagulation is used, the benefit of prophylactic-dose LMWH over prophylactic-dose UFH is uncertain.	IIb BR
In ischemic stroke, elastic compression stockings should not be used.	III* BR
Depression Screening	
Administration of a structured depression inventory is recommended to routinely screen for poststroke depression, but the optimal timing of screening is uncertain.	I BNR
Patients diagnosed with poststroke depression should be treated with antidepressants in the absence of contraindications and closely monitored to verify effectiveness.	I BR
Other	
Routine use of prophylactic antibiotics has not been shown to be beneficial.	III BR

Routine placement of indwelling bladder catheters should not be performed because of the associated risk of catheter-associated urinary tract infections.	III* CLD
During hospitalization and inpatient rehabilitation, regular skin assessments are recommended with objective scales of risk such as the Braden scale.	I CLD
It is recommended to minimize or eliminate skin friction, to minimize skin pressure, to provide appropriate support surfaces, to avoid excessive moisture, and to maintain adequate nutrition and hydration to prevent skin breakdown. Regular turning, good skin hygiene, and use of specialized mattresses, wheelchair cushions, and seating are recommended until mobility returns.	I CLD
It is reasonable for patients and families with stroke to be directed to palliative care resources as appropriate. Caregivers should ascertain and include patient-centered preferences in decision making, especially during prognosis formation and considering interventions or limitations in care.	IIa CED
Rehabilitation	
It is recommended that early rehabilitation for hospitalized stroke patients be provided in environments with organized, interprofessional stroke care.	I A
It is recommended that stroke survivors receive rehabilitation at an intensity commensurate with anticipated benefit and tolerance.	I BNR
High-dose, very early mobilization within 24 hours of stroke onset should not be performed because it can reduce the odds of a favorable outcome at 3 months.	III* BR
It is recommended that all individuals with stroke be provided a formal assessment of their activities of daily living and instrumental activities of daily living, communication abilities, and functional mobility before discharge from acute care hospitalization and the findings be incorporated into the care transition and the discharge planning process.	I BNR
A functional assessment by a clinician with expertise in rehabilitation is recommended for patients with an acute stroke with residual functional deficits.	I CLD
The effectiveness of fluoxetine or other selective serotonin reuptake Inhibitors to enhance motor recovery is not well established.	IIb CLD
5. In-Hospital Management of AIS: Treatment of Acute Complications	
Cerebellar and Cerebral Edema	
Ventriculostomy is recommended in the treatment of obstructive hydrocephalus after a cerebellar infarct. Concomitant or subsequent	I CLD

decompressive craniectomy may or may not be necessary on the basis of factors such as infarct size, neurological condition, degree of brainstem compression, and effectiveness of medical management	
Decompressive suboccipital craniectomy with dural expansion should be performed in patients with cerebellar infarction causing neurological deterioration from brainstem compression despite maximal medical therapy. When deemed safe and indicated, obstructive hydrocephalus should be treated concurrently with ventriculostomy.	I BNR
When considering decompressive suboccipital craniectomy for cerebellar infarction, it may be reasonable to inform family members that the outcome after cerebellar infarct can be good after sub-occipital craniectomy.	IIb CLD
Patients with large territorial supratentorial infarctions are at high risk for complicating brain edema and increased intracranial pressure. Discussion of care options and possible outcomes should take place quickly with patients (if possible) and caregivers. Medical professionals and caregivers should ascertain and include patient-centered preferences in shared decision making, especially during prognosis formation and considering interventions or limitations in care.	I CEO
Patients with major infarctions are at high risk for complicating brain edema. Measures to lessen the risk of edema and close monitoring of the patient for signs of neurological worsening during the first days after stroke are recommended. Early transfer of patients at risk for malignant brain edema to an institution with neurosurgical expertise should be considered.	I CLD
In patients ≤ 60 years of age with unilateral MCA infarctions who deteriorate neurologically within 48 hours despite medical therapy, decompressive craniectomy with dural expansion is reasonable because it reduces mortality by close to 50%, with 55% of the surgical survivors achieving moderate disability (able to walk) or better (mRS score 2 or 3) and 18% achieving independence (mRS score 2) at 12 months.	IIa A
In patients >60 years of age with unilateral MCA infarctions who deteriorate neurologically within 48 hours despite medical therapy, decompressive craniectomy with dural expansion may be considered because it reduces mortality by close to 50%, with 11% of the surgical survivors achieving moderate disability (able to walk [mRS score 3]) and none achieving independence (mRS score ≤ 2) at 12 months.	IIb BR
Although the optimal trigger for decompressive craniectomy is unknown, it is reasonable to use a decrease in level of consciousness attributed to brain swelling as selection criteria.	IIa A
Use of osmotic therapy for patients with clinical deterioration from cerebral swelling associated with cerebral infarction is reasonable.	IIa CLD
Use of brief moderate hyperventilation (Pco2 target 30–34 mm Hg) is a	IIa

reasonable treatment for patients with acute severe neurological decline from brain swelling as a bridge to more definitive therapy.	CEO
Hypothermia or barbiturates in the setting of ischemic cerebral or cerebellar swelling are not recommended.	III BR
Because of a lack of evidence of efficacy and the potential to increase the risk of infectious complications, corticosteroids (in conventional or large doses) should not be administered for the treatment of cerebral edema and increased intracranial pressure complicating ischemic stroke.	III* A
Seizures	
Recurrent seizures after stroke should be treated in a manner similar to when they occur with other acute neurological conditions, and anti-seizure drugs should be selected based upon specific patient characteristics.	I CLD
Prophylactic use of anti-seizure drugs is not recommended.	III BR
6. In-Hospital Institution of Secondary Prevention: Evaluation	
Brain Imaging	
Routine use of brain MRI in all patients with AIS is not cost-effective and is not recommended for initial diagnosis or to plan subsequent treatment.	III BNR
In some patients with AIS, the use of MRI might be considered to provide additional information for initial diagnosis or to plan subsequent treatment, although the effect on outcomes is uncertain.	IIb CEO
Vascular Imaging	
For patients with nondisabling (mRS score 0–2) AIS in the carotid territory who are candidates for CEA or stenting, noninvasive imaging of the cervical vessels should be performed routinely within 24 hours of admission	I BNR
In patients with AIS, routine noninvasive imaging by means of CTA or MRA of the intracranial vasculature to determine the presence of intracranial arterial stenosis or occlusion is not recommended to plan subsequent secondary preventive treatment.	III A
In some patients with AIS, noninvasive imaging by means of CTA or MRA of the intracranial vasculature to provide additional information to plan subsequent secondary preventive treatment may be reasonable, although the effect on outcomes is uncertain.	IIb CEO
Cardiac Evaluation	
Cardiac monitoring is recommended to screen for atrial fibrillation and other potentially serious cardiac arrhythmias that would necessitate	I BNR

emergency cardiac interventions. Cardiac monitoring should be performed for at least the first 24 hours.	
The clinical benefit of prolonged cardiac monitoring to detect atrial fibrillation after AIS is uncertain.	IIb BR
In some patients with AIS, prolonged cardiac monitoring to provide additional information to plan subsequent secondary preventive treatment may be reasonable, although the effect on outcomes is uncertain.	IIb CEO
Routine use of echocardiography in all patients with AIS to plan subsequent secondary preventive treatment is not cost-effective and is not recommended.	III BNR
In selected patients with AIS, echocardiography to provide additional information to plan subsequent secondary preventive treatment may be reasonable.	IIb BR
Glucose	
After AIS, it is reasonable to screen all patients for diabetes mellitus with testing of fasting plasma glucose, hemoglobin A1c, or an oral glucose tolerance test. Choice of test and timing should be guided by clinical judgment and recognition that acute illness may temporarily perturb measures of plasma glucose. In general, hemoglobin A1c may be more accurate than other screening tests in the immediate post-event period.	IIa CEO
Cholesterol	
Routine measurement of blood cholesterol levels in all patients with ischemic stroke presumed to be of atherosclerotic origin who are not already taking a high-intensity statin is not recommended.	III BR
Measurement of blood cholesterol levels in patients with ischemic stroke presumed to be of atherosclerotic origin who are already taking an optimized regimen of statin therapy may be useful for identifying patients who would be candidates for outpatient proprotein convertase subtilisin/kexin type 9 inhibitor treatment to reduce the risk of subsequent cardiovascular death, MI, or stroke.	IIb BR
Other Tests for Secondary Prevention	
Baseline troponin assessment is recommended in patients presenting with AIS but should not delay initiation of IV tPA or mechanical thrombectomy.	I CLD
Routine screening for hyperhomocysteinemia among patients with a recent ischemic stroke is not indicated.	III CEO
The usefulness of screening for thrombophilic states in patients with ischemic stroke is unknown.	IIb CLD
Anticoagulation might be considered in patients who are found to have abnormal findings on coagulation testing after an initial ischemic stroke,	IIb CLD

depending on the abnormality and the clinical circumstances.	
Routine testing for antiphospholipid antibodies is not recommended for patients with ischemic stroke who have no other manifestations of the antiphospholipid syndrome and who have an alternative explanation for their ischemic event, such as atherosclerosis, carotid stenosis, or atrial fibrillation.	III CLD
Routine screening of patients with recent ischemic stroke for obstructive sleep apnea (OSA) is not recommended.	III BR
Antithrombotic Treatment	
For patients with non-cardioembolic AIS, the use of antiplatelet agents rather than oral anticoagulation is recommended to reduce the risk of recurrent stroke and other cardiovascular events.	I A
For patients who have a non-cardioembolic AIS while taking aspirin, increasing the dose of aspirin or switching to an alternative antiplatelet agent for additional benefit in secondary stroke prevention is not well established.	IIb BR
For patients who have a non-cardioembolic AIS while taking antiplatelet therapy, switching to warfarin is not beneficial for secondary stroke prevention.	III BR
For early secondary prevention in patients with non-cardioembolic AIS, the selection of an antiplatelet agent should be individualized on the basis of patient risk factor profiles, cost, tolerance, relative known efficacy of the agents, and other clinical characteristics.	I CEO
For patients with a history of ischemic stroke, atrial fibrillation, and coronary artery disease, the usefulness of adding antiplatelet therapy to oral anticoagulants is uncertain for purposes of reducing the risk of ischemic cardiovascular and cerebrovascular events. Unstable angina and coronary artery stenting represent special circumstances in which management may warrant dual antiplatelet/oral anticoagulation.	IIb CD
For most patients with an AIS in the setting of atrial fibrillation, it is reasonable to initiate oral anticoagulation within 4 to 14 days after the onset of neurological symptoms.	IIa BNR
For patients with AIS and hemorrhagic transformation, initiation or continuation of antiplatelet or anticoagulation therapy may be considered, depending on the specific clinical scenario and underlying indication.	IIb BNR
For patients with AIS and extracranial carotid or vertebral arterial dissection, treatment with either antiplatelet or anticoagulant therapy for 3 to 6 months may be reasonable.	IIb BR
For patients with AIS and extracranial carotid or vertebral arterial dissection who have definite recurrent cerebral ischemic events despite medical therapy, the value of EVT (stenting) is not well established.	IIb CLD

Statins	
Among patients already taking statins at the time of onset of ischemic stroke, continuation of statin therapy during the acute period is reasonable.	IIa BR
High-intensity statin therapy should be initiated or continued as first-line therapy in women and men ≤75 years of age who have clinical ASCVD*, unless contraindicated. *Clinical ASCVD includes acute coronary syndromes, history of MI, stable or unstable angina, coronary or other arterial revascularization, stroke, TIA, or peripheral arterial disease presumed to be of atherosclerotic origin.	I A
In individuals with clinical ASCVD* in whom high-intensity statin therapy would otherwise be used, when high-intensity statin therapy is contraindicated or when characteristics predisposing to statin-associated adverse effects are present, moderate-intensity statin should be used as the second option if tolerated.	I A
In individuals with clinical ASCVD* >75 years of age, it is reasonable to evaluate the potential for ASCVD risk-reduction benefits and for adverse effects and drug–drug interactions and to consider patient preferences when initiating a moderate- or high-intensity statin. It is reasonable to continue statin therapy in those who are tolerating it.	IIb CEO
Patients with ischemic stroke and other comorbid ASCVD should be otherwise managed according to the 2013 ACC/AHA cholesterol guidelines, which include lifestyle modification, dietary recommendations, and medication recommendations.	I A
For patients with an AIS who qualify for statin treatment, in-hospital initiation of statin therapy is reasonable.	IIa CLD
Carotid Revascularization	
When revascularization is indicated for secondary prevention in patients with minor, nondisabling stroke (mRS score 0–2), it is reasonable to perform the procedure between 48 hours and 7 days of the index event rather than delay treatment if there are no contraindications to early revascularization.	IIa BNR
Smoking Cessation Intervention	
Healthcare providers should strongly advise every patient with AIS who has smoked in the past year to quit.	I CEO
Counseling, nicotine products, and oral smoking cessation medications are effective in helping smokers to quit.	I A
For smokers with an AIS, in-hospital initiation of high-intensity behavioral therapies is reasonable.	IIa BR
For smokers with an AIS, in-hospital initiation of varenicline might be	IIb BR

considered.	
For smokers with an AIS, in-hospital initiation of interventions that incorporate both pharmacotherapy and behavioral support might be considered.	IIb BR
It is reasonable to advise patients after ischemic stroke to avoid second-hand (passive) tobacco smoke.	IIa BNR
Stroke Education	
Patient education about stroke is recommended. Patients should be provided with information, advice, and the opportunity to talk about the impact of the illness on their lives.	I CEO

References

1. *Scientific Rationale for the Inclusion and Exclusion Criteria for Intravenous TPA in Acute Ischemic A Stroke Statement for Healthcare Professionals From the American Heart Association/American Stroke Association.* Bart M. Demaerschalk, MD, MSc, FRCPC, FAHA, Chair, Dawn O. Kleindorfer, MD, FAHA, Vice-Chair and Opeolu M. Adeoye, MD, MS, FAHA. s.l. : Stroke, 2015, Vol. 47.
2. *Indications for thrombectomy in acute ischemic stroke from emergent large vessel occlusion (ELVO): report of the SNIS Standards and Guidelines Committee.* Maxim Mokin, 1 Sameer A Ansari, Ryan A McTaggart. s.l. : J NeuroIntervent Surg, 2019.
3. *2018 Guidelines for the Early Management of Patients With Acute Ischemic Stroke: A Guideline for Healthcare Professionals From the American Heart Association/American Stroke Association.* William J. Powers, Alejandro A. Rabinstein , Teri Ackerson ,. s.l. : Stroke, 2018, Vol. 49.

11

Neuro-Angiography Suite and Patient Management During EVT

There are no established guidelines on how to run neuro-angiography (biplane) suite (NAS) and how to manage stroke patient during EVT. Most of the suggestions and recommendations presented here are from author's experience. This chapter will first review the components (equipment and tools) that every NAS should be equipped with, then discuss qualifications and structure of neurointerventional team, and responsibilities of nurses and technologists during EVT.

▪ Neuro-angiography suite

Neuro-angiography suite (NAS) (Figure 11.1) is where endovascular procedures are performed on patients with cerebrovascular diseases that are amenable to EVT. These procedures include catheter angiography, intraarterial (IA) thrombectomy, cerebral aneurysm and AVM embolization, carotid artery stenting (CAS), and many other head and neck vascular procedures. The NA (biplane) machine has the ability to perform high definition fluoroscopic and digital subtraction angiography (DSA) images in two projections simultaneously.

Biplane angiography machine should ideally have DSA capability, high-resolution image intensifier, and imaging chain, digital subtraction imaging (1,024 × 1,024 matrix is ideal). Road map fluoroscopy capabilities with and without simultaneous live unsubtracted imaging are also required. A technologist must document fluoroscopy time, and dosimetry should be used. Biplane and 3-D angiography are essential, and angiography equipment with built-in CT capability tools for stroke interventional procedures are strongly recommended [(1)].

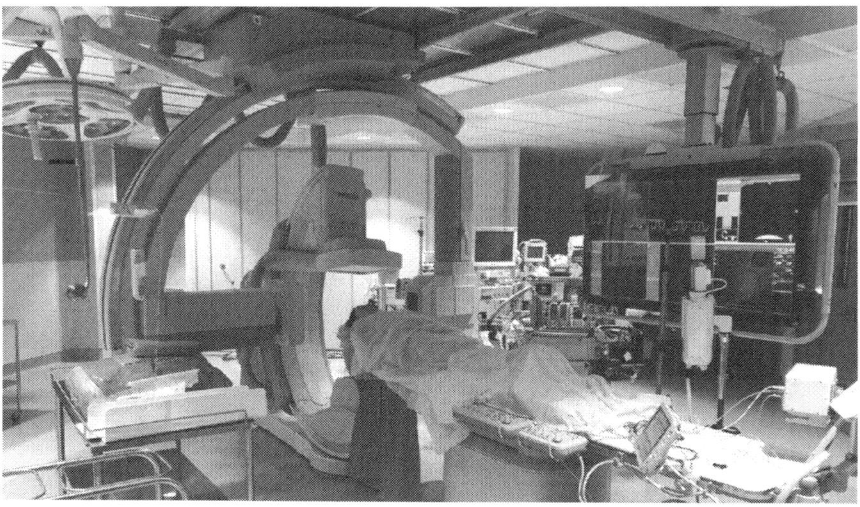

Figure 11.1. Neuroangiography suite with biplane angiography machine, anesthesia machine, high definition screen and tools table.

This type of capability is critical when performing diagnostic or interventional work on the very complex and delicate cerebrovascular bed.

The NAS should have its own anesthesia machine (including necessary hook ups), automated medication dispensing system, tools table (Figure 11.2) and enough storage space for neurointerventional tools. The location of NAS should be situated in close proximity to emergency room, CT suite, MRI suite and Neuro Critical Care Unit (NCCU) to enable efficient workflow and collaboration among different disciplines across the different departments. To ensure timely EVT for acute stroke patient, NAS should be dedicated to the neurointerventional team. Also, postprocedural unit should have enough beds based on volume treated every day. This unit should be in close proximity to NAS.

Neurointerventional tools

Neurointerventional tools are categorized into access tools, interventional tools and ancillary tools. Access tools include access sheaths, diagnostic and guiding catheters, and hemostatic tools.

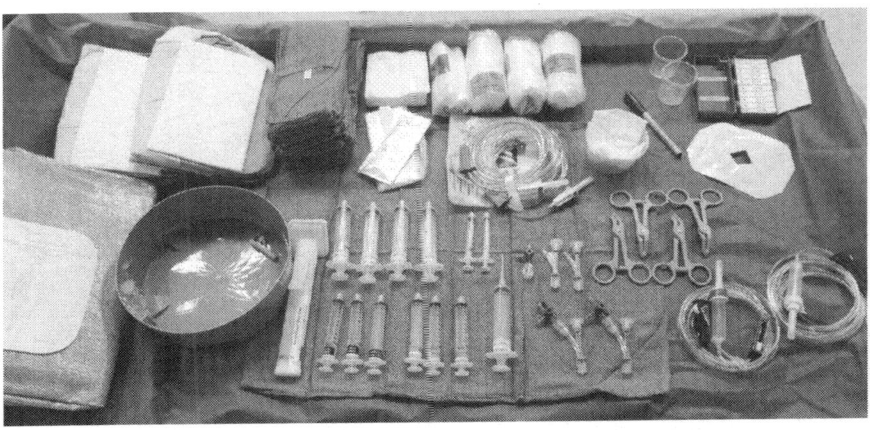

Figure 11.2. Example of basic set up for neurointerventional case.

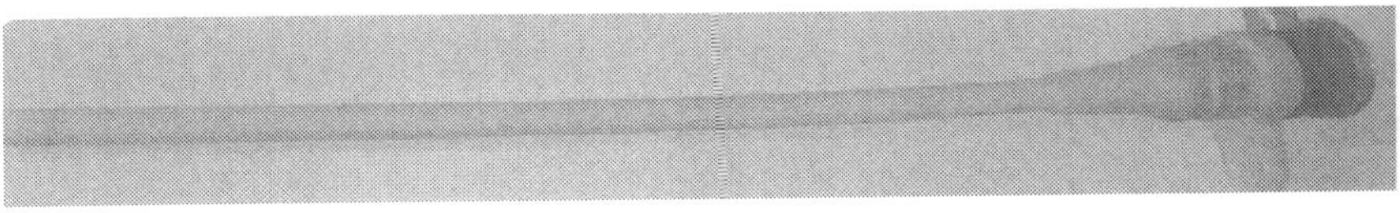

Figure 11.3. An example of a short access sheath.

Access sheath

Access sheath (Figure 11.3) is a short catheter that is placed in femoral artery or radial artery and remains stationary after placement. It is equipped with one-way valve that allows diagnostic or guiding catheters to pass into the artery without needing to go through skin and arterial wall when moved or replaced with a different catheter. They are usually measured in French system and they range from 4 to 9 French gauge. Each size allows catheter of equal or lower gauge to pass. These sheaths come in different lengths (10, 15, 25, 30, 45, 60, 70, 90 cm. etc.) except for the 4 French sheath that typically comes in 10 cm length.

Diagnostic/guiding catheter

Diagnostic and guiding catheters are long catheters used to access the target artery and enables the interventionist to infuse contrast medium directly to obtain high definition picture of the vessel while the contrast is carried by blood flow through vasculature. They have different tip shapes, sizes and lengths. The diagnostic catheter has smaller inner lumen and usually comes in 4 and 5 French gauge. The most common tip shapes are straight, angled, curved (SIM 1 and SIM 2), and C -shape (head hunter). The length of these catheters varies between 60 and 120 cm.

Guiding catheters have larger inner lumen and variety of gauges such as 5, 6, and 7 French. The guiding catheter's inner lumen diameter is larger than the respective same-sized diagnostic catheter. The length ranges from 80 to 110 cm. There is a smaller variety of shapes (straight, angled, SIM) compared to diagnostic catheters. There are special guiding catheters that are used as sheath and guiding catheter at the same time due to uniquely engineered transitional shaft design and they are usually used in EVT for stroke and carotid artery stenting.

Diagnostic and guiding catheters need *guiding wires* that help navigate the catheter into its target without injuring the vessels that carry the catheter. These wires come in different sizes (0.018", 0.025", 0.035", 0.038"), length (120-260 cm), coating (usually hydrophilic) and softness (standard, stiff).

Hemostatic tools

Hemostatic tools are also called vascular closure devices (VCD). They are used at the conclusion of the intervention to secure puncture side and prevent bleeding. They are usually used in healthy femoral artery when there is concern of bleeding due to the use of anticoagulation or dual antiplatelets and concern about patient cooperation with post procedural puncture site precautions. There are three main categories: collagen-based, clip-based, and suture-based devices. There is not enough data to favor one over another. They are safe overall and effective in achieving quick hemostasis. Manual compression is still favored when repeated femoral artery puncture is planned and if the femoral artery is diseased.

Interventional tools

Interventional tools are the tools that are used to access the cerebral vascular lesion through the access sheath and guiding catheter in concentric fashion (Figure 11.4). Interventional tools are divided into non-implantable and implantable. Non-implantable tools include microcatheters, microwires, aspiration catheters, micro balloons (compliant and non-complaint), non-detachable cranial stent (stentriever), and devices that are used to retrieve broken devices from vasculature. Implantable tools included, detachable micro coils, intracranial stents, flow diverters, nBCA glue, Onyx and intra-aneurysmal devices.

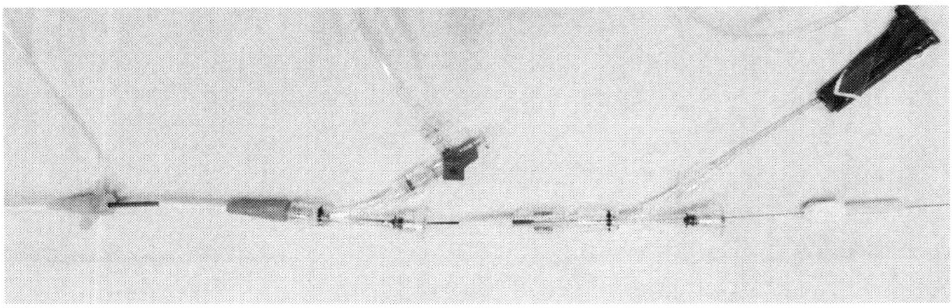

Figure 11.4. The sheath, guiding catheter, micro-catheter and microwires are coaxially connected to help access the target lesion.

Micro catheters (Figure 11.5) have different gauges (1.5, 1.7, 1.9, 2.3, 2.5, 2.7, 2.8 French), lengths (105-160 cm) and shapes (straight, angled, C-shape, S- shape, etc.). ***Microwires*** have different sizes (0.08", 0.010", 0.014", 0.017) softness and lengths (180-300 cm). Micro wire and micro catheter are advanced as one unit in the intracranial vasculature (Figure 11.6).

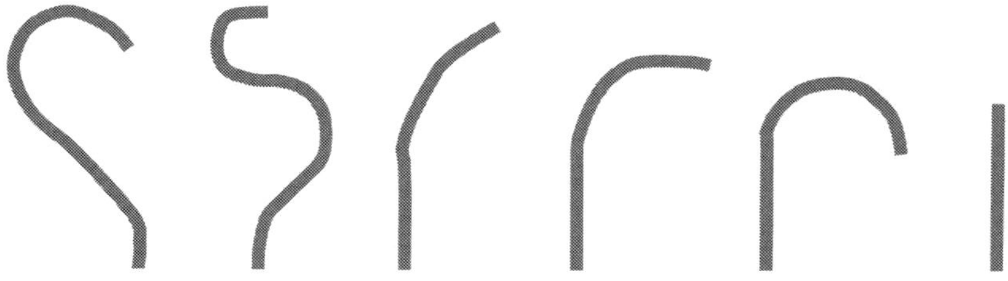

Figure 11.5. Different shapes of microcatheter tip (C, S, 45-degree, 90-degree, J shape and straight from right to left).

Aspiration catheters are microcatheters that are reinforced to prevent collapse with negative pressure and are used mainly in ischemic stroke to aspirate clots from brain.

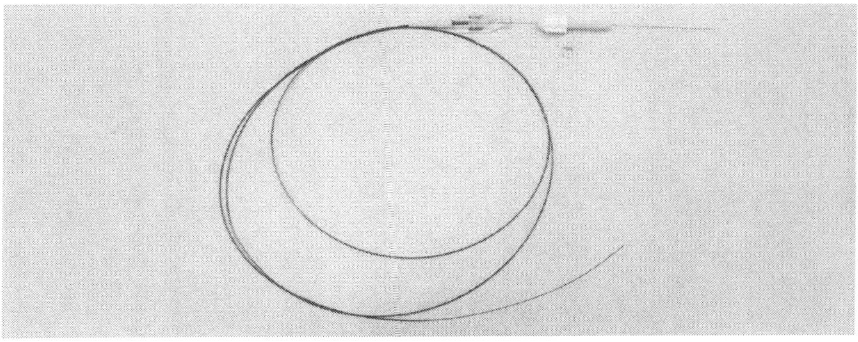

Figure 11.6. Example of microcatheter with microwire within the catheter.

Micro coils (Figure 11.7) are used to embolize cerebral aneurysms and there is a large collection of sizes, designs, diameters (1-20mm), softness and length (1-50cm).

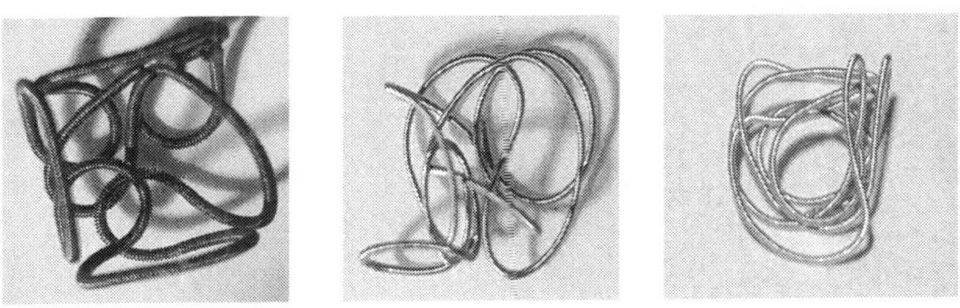

Figure 11.7. Example of micro coils.

Compliant micro balloons (Figure 11.8) come in different sizes and designs and are used for balloon-assist coiling, Onyx infusion, balloon occlusion tests (BTO) and for emergent arterial hemostasis. On the other hand, ***non-compliant micro balloons*** (Figure 11.9) are used for angioplasty and are made in different sizes and designs.

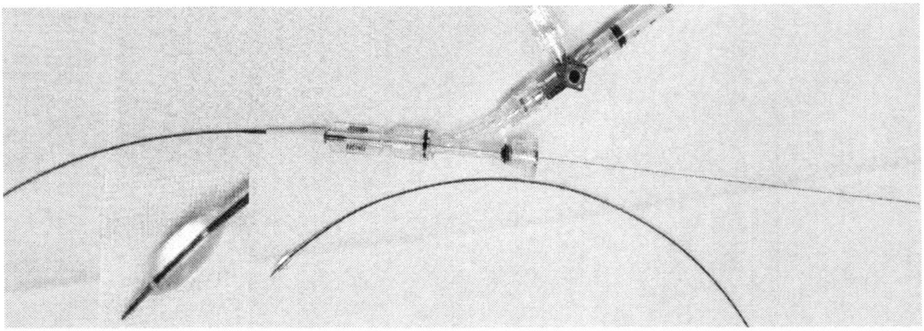

Figure 11.8. Example of micro balloon used for balloon asset coiling.

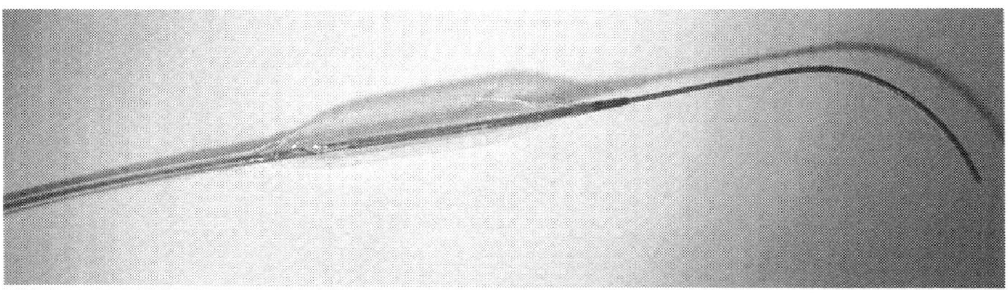

Figure 11.9. Example of micro balloon used for balloon angioplasty in intracranial arterial system.

Intracranial stent are three types based on diseases they are designed to treat: ***atherosclerosis stent*** to treat intracranial stenosis and ***aneurysmal stents*** (Figure 11.10) are used to assist micro coils during cerebral aneurysm embolization. ***Flow diverter*** (FD) (Figure 11.11) can be considered a stent; however, unlike other aneurysmal stents, it is used to divert flow away from the aneurysm without using micro coils to fill the aneurysm. nBCA (adhesive) and Onyx (cohesive) are designed to treat arteriovenous malformations and fistulas.

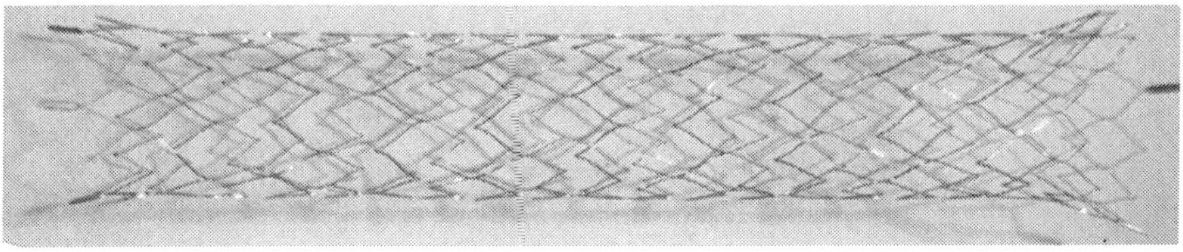

Figure 11.10. An example of an aneurysmal stent that assists coiling.

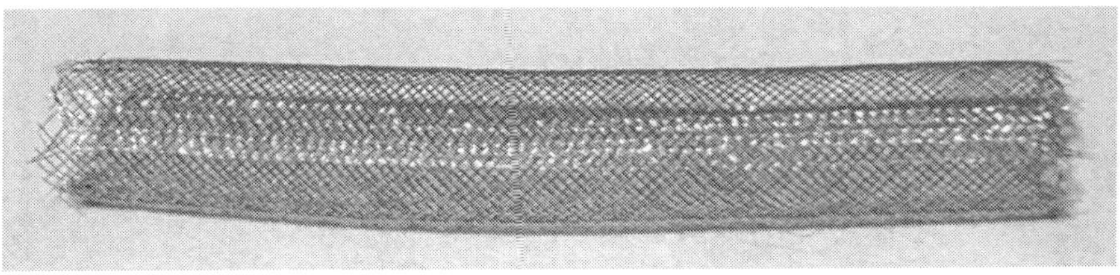

Figure 11.11. An example of flow diverting stent.

▪ Neurointerventional team qualifications & expectations

Neurointerventional team consists of neuro-interventionist, neurointerventional technical / administrative director, technologists and nurses. Due to advancement of management of neurointerventional disease and evolution of sophisticated options, neurointerventionist performing EVT should be fellowship trained in neurointerventional procedures.

Neurointerventional technical/administrative director

The technical / administrative director works in conjunction with the medical director to ensure quality control of the stroke interventional suite. The administrative director should oversee control of patient scheduling, equipment maintenance, budget preparation, monitoring radiation doses, organization of conferences for laboratory personnel, and regular reports on laboratory activity. The director must work closely with the medical director to establish basic standards for personnel, maintenance, quality assurance, quality improvement, continuing education, and any financial decisions that directly impact the operations of the stroke intervention laboratory [(2)].

Interventional technologist(s)

A variety of knowledgeable technical personnel may be required for the sake of efficiency in operating a stroke interventional laboratory, and one person is unlikely to possess all different expertise. At least one technologist, preferably a certified radiological technologist, should be skilled in radiographic and angiographic imaging principles and techniques. This technologist should be experienced in the proper performance of X-ray generators, cine pulse systems, image intensification, automatic film processing, pressure injection systems, video systems, and cine cameras. He or she in conjunction with radiological service engineers should be responsible for routine care and maintenance of radiological equipment. The basic ability to troubleshoot equipment in the stroke interventional laboratory is advantageous. This technologist, in cooperation with radiation physicist, must monitor radiation safety techniques for both the patient and laboratory personnel. Immediate availability of radiological engineer in the event of the equipment failure is highly desirable [(2)].

Interventional nurse(s)

The utility of nursing personnel may vary in type and number in the stroke interventional laboratory, depending on case load and mix, and may include nurse practitioners, registered nurses, licensed vocational or practical nurses, or nursing assistants. In most laboratories, the nursing supervisor is a registered nurse. This nurse must be familiar with all overall function of the laboratory, help set the tone of patient surroundings, and influence the efficiency and safety of procedures. Nursing staff may directly participate in observation, emergency response, and charge the pre and post-procedural holding areas. Nursing staff must assist with hemodynamic and neurological monitoring for regular documentation of vital signs and neurological assessments [(2)].

Anesthesia support

The utility of general anesthesia during stroke interventional procedures has not been validated and remains a topic of controversy. The majority of stroke interventionalists nationally practice conscious sedation or monitored anesthesia for LVO EVT cases unless the patient needs airway protection, in which case general anesthesia is provided. In a fully credentialed stroke interventional laboratory, full anesthesia support must be available for complicated cases during which intubation and sedation is indicated. It is not recommended to practice routine general anesthesia for all patients and must be reviewed by individual cases. Level 1 conscious sedation practices are recommended for stroke interventional procedures, under the supervision of appropriately trained providers [(2)].

Procedure preparation and conduct

Although no rigid protocol is applicable to all laboratories, certain procedural issues, such as premedication, should be addressed. In cases where conscious sedation is required, fixed protocols should be maintained during the procedure. Sterile preparation is mandatory for all vascular access sites. All operators must wear masks, caps, and eye protection to prevent accidental operator contamination [(2)].

Proper procedural technique includes adequate injections of cerebral vasculature, including the aortic arch, and use of multiple views with appropriate radiographic angulation for visualization of the cerebral vascular structures. Patients should have adequate monitoring including hemodynamic monitoring of basic vital signs (blood pressure, heart, rate, respiratory rate, and oxygen saturation) along with frequent neurological checks, which must be documented in flow sheets during the procedure [(2)].

Post-procedural hemostasis may be achieved by several means including manual pressure, mechanical compression devices, or percutaneous closure devices. Patients should be monitored after procedure for hematoma and pseudoaneurysms, and event rates of each method and each device must be tracked (2).

Antiplatelet agents, including aspirin and clopidogrel, do not need to be withheld before cerebral angiography. Warfarin should be discontinued until INR is <1.8, if clinically indicated after a discussion of the risks and benefits with the patient or family. If necessary, warfarin may be reversed with FFP or vitamin K as per pharmacy protocol [(2)].

Brain attack activation protocol for nurses, imaging technologists, anesthesiologists, ED team, and stroke interventionalists

The stroke interventionalists must operate within a structured framework of support staff and services from the EMS, ED, radiology, and stroke interventional laboratory. AIS patients, from the time of first contact in the field by EMS, need to be triaged according to treatment modality, either IV t-PA, stroke intervention, or medical management focused on secondary prevention. In efforts to improve outcomes and reduce mortality in AIS patients, national guidelines, protocols, and algorithms have been developed and organized into a systems operation for facilitating the selection of patients eligible for IV t-PA administration. Fifty-three international trials in the past several decades, including the NINDS and ECASS trials, demonstrate a significant reduction in 3-month mortality and morbidity for stroke patients who undergo recanalization [(2)].

Identifying and establishing criteria for selecting patients ideal for stroke intervention has historically been less straightforward, based on results from trials such as IMS-III and MR-RESCUE. Currently, between the results of the FIRST study, which demonstrates the natural history of stroke to be devastating with nearly 80% of LVO AIS patients either dead or disabled for life if left untreated, and a clear benefit of endovascular revascularization therapies for LVO AIS in several recent landmark trials including the MR-CLEAN trial, there is a paradigm shift. There is an imminent unmet need to create advanced algorithms that facilitate the identification of LVO AIS patients appropriate for stroke interventional procedures from the moment of initial contact with EMS [(2)].

Post-procedural care

All patients should be observed on bed rest during the initial post-procedural period. Depending on the size of the arteriotomy, use of arteriotomy closure devices, anticoagulants or antiplatelet agents, and procedural and disease-specific risk factors, continued bed rest may be required. During the initial post-procedural period, skilled nurses or other trained professionals should periodically monitor the puncture site for hematoma development and the status of the vascular distribution distal to the puncture sites. Monitoring of indwelling arterial sheaths to assure continuous flushing should be performed. Neurologic monitoring is required to detect delayed neurologic deterioration [(2)].

Post-procedural monitoring should be conducted in a manner appropriate to the disease process and anatomic lesion treated. The patient should be monitored for urinary output, renal function, cardiac symptoms, pain, and other indicators of systemic complications. Further laboratory evaluation of hematologic, coagulation, or organ function may be indicated. Appropriate follow-up imaging (radiography of the skull, CT, MR, angiography) should be ordered as indicated [(2)].

The initial ambulation of the patient must be supervised. The operating physician or designee should evaluate the patient's condition after the procedure. Documentation of involvement should consist of entries in the patient's hospital record. The operating physician or designee should be available for continuing care during hospitalization and after discharge [(2)].

Neurointerventional team should be vigilant and well-equipped to assess and treat complications. When discussing the risks of complications, patient should be made aware of puncture site complications, neuroangiography complications, and contrast media-induced nephropathy. These complications may be greater with interventional procedures than for diagnostic neuroangiography because the need for larger or bilateral guide catheters. Dissection of catheterized vessels are reported more frequently during neurointerventional procedures because of more prolonged positioning of generally larger guide catheters [2]. Treating puncture site complications and other complications is highlighted in chapter 12 in the post EVT order set discussion.

References

1. *Basic Neuroangiography: Review of Technique and Perioperative Patient Care.* Sun Ho Ahn, MD, Ethan A. Prince, MD, and Gregory J. Dubel, MD. 3, s.l. : Semin Intervent Radiol, 2013, Vol. 30.

2. *Society of Vascular and Interventional Neurology (SVIN) Stroke Interventional Laboratory Consensus (SILC) Criteria: A 7M Management Approach to Developing a Stroke Interventional Laboratory in the Era of Stroke Thrombectomy for Large Vessel Occlusions.* Tanzila Shams, Osama Zaidat, Dileep Yavagal. 1-2, s.l. : Interv Neurol, 2016, Vol. 5.

12

Management of AIS for First 24 Hours and After IV tPA and EVT

▪ Admission recommendations

The following are recommendations for inpatient management of ischemic stroke and transient ischemic attack (TIA). After receiving the stroke patient, the stroke code team should activate "stroke code order set". After establishing the diagnosis of ischemic stroke and implementing specific treatment, the treating team should determine the most appropriate unit for admission: inpatient stroke unit (ISU) or neuro intensive care unit (NICU).

Admission to NICU

Treating team should admit patient into NICU if following conditions are met:

- o Post IV tPA or EVT.
- o Hemispheric stroke with potential inability to protect airway or decline in level of consciousness (LOC).
- o Basilar artery stroke (due to possible deterioration into coma).
- o Fluctuating symptoms or FIND (Table 3.4, chapter 3) to be able to perform neuro-check every 1-2 hours.

- o Need for IV pressers (BP augmentation due to critical arterial stenosis) or need for IV drugs to control blood pressure or heart rate.

Admission to ISU

Treating team should admit patient into ISU if following conditions are met:

- o Acute stroke symptoms or TIA and not meeting NICU criteria.

After determining the most appropriate unit, treatment team should communicate to the appropriate admitting team to transfer over care. The receiving team should activate appropriate stroke admission order set; "inpatient stroke/TIA order set", "post IV tPA order set", or "NICU stroke order set". After EVT, the neurointerventional team should complete "post procedure order set" immediately after finishing the procedure.

Order sets

Post IV tPA order set

- o No IV heparin, warfarin, DOACs, or antiplatelet drugs during and for 24 hours post infusion of tPA.
- o Head CT or MRI at 24 hours post infusion.
- o Neuro checks and vital signs every 30 minutes for 6 hrs., then every 1 hour for 16 hours, and then per NICU standard of care.
- o If the patient already has an invasive line upon arrival from another hospital (i.e., arterial or central), observe very carefully for bleeding at the site and apply pressure as needed.
- o Maintain IV's already in place (restart only if necessary).
- o Observe changes in neurologic exam and inform team: neurologic deterioration (NIHSS change of > 3), sudden marked changes in vital signs, changes in LOC, nausea, vomiting,

diaphoresis, new headache. Immediately discontinue IV t-PA and notify stroke team.

- Observe for any signs of adverse drug reaction.
- Assess IV/arterial puncture sites, urine, gums, skin, stool, emesis, etc. for bleeding.
- Keep head of bed 30 degrees (preferably lower degree if still within first 24 hours of onset if no risk of aspiration and no increased ICP).
- Bed rest for 24 hours, then increase activity as tolerated.
- Avoid placement of nasogastric (NG) tubes, blood draws, or invasive lines/procedures for 24 hours post infusion, if possible.
- No intramuscular injections.
- Dysphagia screening to be completed and documented prior to anything by mouth using the bedside nurse swallow screen.
- Initiate speech language therapist consult for formal swallow evaluation, as needed, and when patient able to participate.
- Goal systolic blood pressure (SBP) <180 mmHg, diastolic blood pressure (DBP) <105:

SBP 180-230 OR DBP 105-120:

- Nicardipine IV 5 mg give initial dose, then 5 mg/hour IV infusion as initial dose and titrate to desired effect by increasing rate by 2.5 mg/hour every 5 minutes to maximum of 15 mg/hour.
- Labetalol 10 mg IV given over 1-2 minutes; may repeat or double labetalol every 10-20 minutes to maximum dose of 300 mg

SBP >230 OR DBP 121-140:

- Nicardipine IV 5 mg give initial dose, then 5 mg/hour IV infusion as initial dose and titrate to desired effect by increasing rate by 2.5 mg/hour every 5 minutes to maximum of 15 mg/hour.
- Labetalol 10 mg IV given over 1-2 minutes; may repeat or double labetalol every 10 minutes to maximum dose of 300 mg, consider a labetalol drip at 2-8 mg/min.
- If BP is not controlled by labetalol or nicardipine, consider sodium nitroprusside.

DBP >140:

- Sodium nitroprusside 0.5 mcg/kg/min IV infusion initial dose and titrate to desired blood pressure.

Post EVT Order Set

Use same IV tPA order set with additional puncture site precautions:

- Check puncture site (if sheath still in place) for bleeding or hematoma every 30 minutes for 6 hrs., then every 1 hour for 16 hours, and then per NICU standard of care.
- Check puncture site (if sheath is removed) for bleeding or hematoma every 30 minutes for 3 hrs., then every 1 hour for 3 hours, and then per NICU standard of care. Re-apply manual compression (MC) for 30 minutes and external compression device (ECD) if hematoma or bleeding found.
- Remove sheath 24 hours after IV tPA infusion and apply MC for 30 minutes. Use ECD (such as FemStop) if site continues to ooze bleed. Re-apply MC for additional 30 minutes and use ECD afterward.
- It is recommended to keep SBP is < 140 during sheath removal and for 2 hours afterward.
- Obtain STAT INR, PTT, CBC, fibrinogen, type and cross if bleeding continues.
- Call neurointerventional team if bleeding is uncontrollable while maintaining good MC.
- Keep leg straight as long as sheath is in place and for 6 hours after achieving hemostasis using MC or for 3 hours after use of vascular closure device (VCD).

Suspected Hemorrhagic Transformation (HT)

If clinical suspicion of hemorrhagic transformation (HT) (neurological deterioration, new headache, acute hypertension, nausea or vomiting):

- Obtain STAT Head NCCT, INR, PTT, platelet count, fibrinogen, type and cross.

- Prepare for administration of cryoprecipitate or antifibrinolytics (discussed in detail in chapter 13).
- Consider 6-8 units of platelets.

Additional orders

NICU Order Set to Optimize Physiologic Condition

These are additional order sets that may be considered when a patient is admitted to NICU:

- Isotonic fluids for volume restoration. Central venous pressure (CVP) monitoring to guide volume therapy.
- Vasopressors, if necessary, to achieve BP goal.
- Continuous arterial pressure monitoring is recommended to help with close titration of vasoactive medications.
- Central line or PICC line if using or anticipate using vasoactive medication and/or hypertonic saline.
- Monitor electrolytes, blood counts, coagulation status.
- Maintain glucose within normal limits. Use insulin sliding scale titrated to blood glucose 120-160 mg/dL. Use insulin infusion if blood glucose > 180 mg/dL for two consecutive checks.
- Observe for hyponatremia. Administer hypertonic saline as needed.
- Maintain normothermia. If fever, identify source; target work up and antibiotics to possible source(s); use antipyretics (acetaminophen, cooling blankets, ice packs etc) to achieve goals.
- Consider ICP monitoring and/or EVD for patients based on poor neurological status: Glasgow Coma Scale (GCS) score <8 or neurological deterioration with hydrocephalus or any concern for ICP elevation. If EVD placed, ICP goal < 20 with cerebrospinal fluid (CSF) surveillance sampling q 72h by neurosurgery (more frequent if clinically indicated).
- If rapid edema formation is suspected or observed consult neurosurgery service for initial evaluation in preparation for

emergency decompressive craniectomy should it become a therapeutic option.

Orders after 24 hours of IV tPA

- o Initiate venous thromboembolism (VTE) prophylaxis by end of day one, as appropriate, unless contraindicated.
- o Ensure patient is receiving antithrombotics within 24 hours of admission and upon discharge, unless contraindicated.
- o Ensure that patients with atrial fibrillation are receiving anti-coagulation therapy on discharge, unless contraindicated.
- o Initiate peptic ulcer prophylaxis (PUD) if indicated.
- o Obtain lipid profile. Initiate statin to lower LDL if needed.
- o Evaluate need for bowel and bladder training. Maintain regular toileting schedule.
- o Initiate fall and pressure ulcer prevention interventions.

▪ Treatment of complications

While managing stroke patients after IV tPA and /or EVT, treating providers should be familiar with complications related to IV tPA and EVT. This will help anticipate needed care and prepare for the worst by incorporating a more specific therapeutic plan into the above mentioned routinely implemented plan to minimize the negative effect of complications on patient outcome. Also, it is very helpful that treating physicians know what measures were taken during the procedure to treat any procedural complications.

Hemorrhagic Transformation (HT)

The most feared complication of AIS is ICH or hemorrhagic transformation (HT). HT after IV tPA or EVT are classified (according to ECASS 1 and 2 trials) into: hemorrhagic infarction type 1 (HI 1, small petechiae); hemorrhagic infarction type 2 (HI 2, confluent petechiae); parenchymal hematoma type 1 (PH 1, < 30% of the infarcted area); and parenchymal hematoma type 2 (PH 2, > 30% of the infarcted area with significant mass effect). HT can also be extra-ischemic hematoma (distant hematoma from infarcted zone) [(1)].

There are many risk factors for HT in addition to IV tPA and EVT [(2)]:

- o Massive cerebral infarction (and high NIHSS score) is one of the most dangerous factors
- o Involvement of grey matter (cerebral cortex), because of its abundant collateral circulation, which tends to worsen the reperfusion injury
- o Atrial fibrillation (cerebral embolism)
- o Hyperglycemia
- o Lower LDL-C and total cholesterol levels
- o Lower platelet count
- o Poor baseline collaterals

There are no established guidelines for BP management after EVT; however, there is correlation between systolic blood pressure and HT. The higher the peak values of SBP in the first 24 hours after EVT, the worse the functional outcomes at 90 days and greater severity of hemorrhagic complications within 48 hours after EVT [(3)]. Thus, the author suggests keeping SBP 100-160 in the first 24 hours after EVT and this goal can be adjusted to 100-140 if there is puncture site bleeding (and during sheath removal and for 2 hours after sheath removal using MC) or to 140-180 if perfusion at the end of EVT is still compromised or no recanalization is established.

▪ EVT complications [4]

Early recognition of EVT complications is crucial to significantly reduce bad outcome; therefore, the neuro-interventionalist should be familiar with these complications and their management.

Intracerebral Hemorrhage (ICH)

As discussed above, ICH is the most feared complication of EVT. ICH most likely occurs secondary to re-perfusing tissue that has already infarcted. ICH could also be secondary to direct perforation of a vessel by a catheter, microwire, or device. The effect of ICH can be severe, particularly if thrombolytic or antithrombotic agents were used. HT is already discussed in detail above.

Vessel Perforation

In vessel perforation, like any other complication, early recognition and immediate implementation of treatment is of the highest importance. Once perforation is confirmed, any ongoing thrombolytic, antithrombotic, or antiplatelet medication should be stopped immediately, and coagulopathy should be reversed with appropriate agents (discussed in chapter 13). While waiting to initiate reversal strategies, temporary balloon occlusion at the site of perforation might be considered to prevent further bleeding. Sacrificing a vessel in order to stop bleeding may be necessary to save the patient's life. Head NCCT should be obtained immediately to evaluate the size and location of the bleed (this can be done in most NAS) [4].

Patients with a suspected or confirmed ICH should be sent to the neurocritical care unit after immediate resuscitation measures. Blood pressure management is crucial in managing ICH. It is recommended to keep SBP 120-160 mmHg and DBP less than 90 mmHg [4]. If there is no concern about decreased perfusion, the author recommends keeping SBP 100-140 mmHg.

It is very important to differentiate between ICH and extravasation of contrast (which is considered more benign). Extravasation may occur because of the impaired blood–brain barrier. MRI is particularly useful in differentiating between a hemorrhage and extravasation of contrast from blood–brain barrier disruption. The susceptibility artifact (on T1 and T2) generated by the different hemoglobin degradation products is detected very well by MRI. Conversely, iodinated contrast does not cause susceptibility artifacts and therefore is not detected by the MRI [4].

Vessel perforation will likely cause SAH. Prevention, early recognition, and treatment for vasospasm should be considered. Ventriculostomy placement may be indicated with hydrocephalus on CT scan, suspected elevated intracranial pressures, or when intracranial pressure needs to be monitored and controlled. Early surgical decompression and prevention of cerebral edema may be useful in particular for ICH in the posterior fossa [4].

Arterial Dissection

Endovascular intervention can cause iatrogenic intracranial and extracranial dissection (~0.4%). Although iatrogenic dissection may be benign in many cases, it can also result in significant neurologic deficits. Angioplasty or stenting could be considered for a flow-limiting dissection or to access a distal clot through a dissection. If the dissection does not compromise the blood flow or the patient's neurologic status, then medical treatment with antithrombotic or antiplatelet agents can be considered [4]. The author recommends SBP 100-140 mmHg especially if dissection is intracranial and no compromised perfusion in the territory of dissected vessel.

In situ Thrombosis

In situ thrombosis and clot formation associated with endovascular therapy are significant complications and account for a large proportion of worsening neurologic status associated with EVT. Clot formation and thrombosis are likely related to the induction of the coagulation process and platelet activation, as well as the limited blood flow induced by interventional devices in areas where blood flow may already be compromised by the acute stroke. A continuous infusion of heparinized normal saline, which flushes out the system, is important to prevent thrombosis. To treat in situ thrombosis, we suggest giving heparin boluses to optimize anticoagulation. Adding a small dose of a glycoprotein IIb/IIIa inhibitor might be considered. If these treatments fail, then mechanical removal of thrombus may be necessary [4].

Air Emboli

Although air emboli during EVT are rarely symptomatic, they were reported to account for almost 0.08% of significant neurologic deficits in a large review of nearly 4,500 patients. The source of the air emboli might be the arterial flushed line or suddenly applied negative pressure causing air to enter the catheter. The best approach to avoid air emboli is to meticulously and gently prep and flush the catheters and the devices to remove the air bubbles, and to minimize the number of microcatheter runs. If air emboli result in symptomatic deficits, then use of 100% oxygen or a hyperbaric chamber to treat those complications may be considered [4].

Distal Emboli

The risk of distal migration of a clot is a concern during manipulation to retrieve a clot. The clot may migrate more distally to another single branch or might break into small clots and cause multiple distal emboli in multiple smaller branches. The interventionalist at this time might consider changing the treatment strategy, depending on the new locations of the clots. If the clot is proximal, recanalization can be achieved with aspiration catheter. If the clot is more distal or in multiple branches, thrombolytics may be considered [(4)].

Vasospasm

Catheter and wire manipulation can result in arterial vasospasm. Transluminal angioplasty and IA vasodilator administration have been the mainstay of endovascular vasospasm treatment. Calcium channel blockers such as nicardipine and verapamil have also been shown to improve vasospasm [(4)].

Carotid Cavernous Fistula

Carotid cavernous fistula usually results from a direct wire perforation during a revascularization manipulation. Rarely, it results from an angioplasty. Multiple strategies have been used to treat the fistula, including stent placement or a stent-assisted coil occlusion of the fistula. Onyx (vinyl alcohol copolymer) embolization into the cavernous sinus has been prescribed, either with a direct transorbital access or via a transvenous access. Onyx embolization can also be achieved intra-arterially into the cavernous sinus through the perforation if the interventionalist maintains access after the perforation [(4)].

References

1. *Hemorrhagic Transformation of Ischemic Brain TissueAsymptomatic or Symptomatic?* Christian Berger, MD, Marco Fiorelli, MD and Thorsten Steiner, MD. s.l. : Stroke, 2001, Vols. 32: 1330-1335.
2. *Hemorrhagic transformation after cerebral infarction: current concepts and challenges.* Jie Zhang, Yi Yang Huijie Sun, Yingqi Xing. 8, s.l. : Ann Transl Med, 2014, Vol. 2.
3. *Systolic Blood Pressure Within 24 Hours After Thrombectomy for Acute Ischemic Stroke Correlates With Outcome.* Eva A. Mistry, MBBS, Akshitkumar M. Mistry, MD, Mohammad Obadah Nakawah, MD. 5, s.l. : J Am Heart Assoc, 2017, Vol. 6.
4. *Complications of endovascular therapy foracute ischemic stroke and proposedmanagement approach.* Ziad Darkhabani, MD, Thanh Nguyen, MD, Marc A. Lazzaro, MD. 1, s.l. : Neurology, 2012, Vol. 79.

13

Management of ICH & Anticoagulation Reversal

Rapid diagnosis and implementation of emergency treatment for ICH (similar to ischemic stroke) is of the highest importance, because early deterioration is common in the first few hours after ICH onset. The provider should suspect hemorrhagic stroke if the patient presents, in addition to neurological deficit, with vomiting, SBP >220 mm Hg, severe headache, coma or decreased level of consciousness, and when symptoms progress over minutes or hours. One important aspect of ICH is that more than 20% of patients will experience a decrease in the Glasgow Coma Scale (GCS) of 2 or more points between the prehospital EMS assessment and the initial evaluation in the ED. Furthermore, another 15% to 23% of patients demonstrate continued deterioration within the first hours after hospital arrival [(1)].

Please refer to table 10.2 for strength and level of evidence while reading guidelines and recommendations.

▪ Prehospital management

Most of the time, EMS providers are not able to distinguish acute ischemic stroke (AIS) from intracerebral hemorrhage (ICH).

This why the author recommends maintaining SBP 90-180 mmHg (preferably 140-160 mmHg) during transportation in ambulance to prevent hematoma expansion or aneurysm re-rupture in case symptoms were related to ICH or SAH.

It is equally important to transport the patient to closest stroke center that is equipped with acute stroke treatment. Similar to ischemic stroke, EMS providers should obtain a focused history regarding the timing of symptom onset (or LKW); medical history, medications, and drug use; and contact information for family. EMS providers should provide advanced notice to the ED, so stroke algorithms can be triggered, and stroke code team alerted. Advanced notice significantly shortens time to CT. Prehospital CT in stroke ambulance may allow for triage to an appropriate hospital and initiation of ICH-specific therapy [(1)].

▪ ED management

If an ED is not prepared to manage ICH (due to lack of neurology, neuroradiology, neurosurgery, and critical care capability), there should be a plan for rapid transfer to a center where such services are available. Triaging ICH is very similar to triaging ischemic stroke and stroke code team should be contacted immediately to guide diagnostic and therapeutic emergent plan. ICH patients are more often sleepier on initial presentation, and this may diminish the utility of the NIHSS. Numerous grading scales exist specifically for ICH [(1)]. ICH score is explained in chapter 2, Table 2.1.

After establishing diagnosis, emergency providers should arrange for rapid admission to stroke unit or NICU (or transfer to nearest capable center) and initiate early management. Lowering blood pressure and reversal of coagulopathy should be initiated in the ED immediately after establishing the diagnosis [(1)] (follow protocol in Figure 7.4 in chapter 7).

Table 13.2. Essential components of intracerebral hemorrhage (ICH) work up in Emergency Department.

Integral Components of the History, Physical Examination, and Workup of the Patient with ICH in the Emergency Department (1)	
History	
Time of symptom onset (or time the patient was last normal) Initial symptoms and progression of symptoms	
Vascular risk factors	History of stroke or ICH, hypertension, diabetes mellitus, and smoking
Medications	Anticoagulant drugs, antiplatelet agents, antihypertensive medications, stimulants (including diet pills), sympathomimetic drugs
Recent trauma or surgery	Carotid endarterectomy or carotid stenting, because ICH may be related to hyperperfusion after such procedures
Dementia	Associated with amyloid angiopathy
Alcohol or illicit drug use	Cocaine and other sympathomimetic drugs are associated with ICH, stimulants
Seizures	
Liver disease	May be associated with coagulopathy
Cancer and hematologic disorders	May be associated with coagulopathy
Physical examination	
Vital signs	
A general physical examination focusing on the head, heart, lungs, abdomen, and extremities	
A focused neurological examination	A structured examination such as the National Institutes of Health Stroke Scale can be completed in minutes and provides a quantification that allows easy communication of the severity of the event

	to other caregivers. GCS score is similarly well known and easily computed.
Serum and urine tests	
Complete blood count, electrolytes, blood urea nitrogen and creatinine, and glucose	Higher serum glucose is associated with worse outcome
Prothrombin time (with INR) and an activated partial thromboplastin time	Warfarin-related hemorrhages are associated with an increased hematoma volume, greater risk of expansion, and increased morbidity and mortality
Cardiac-specific troponin	Elevated troponin levels are associated with worse outcome
Toxicology screen to detect cocaine and other sympathomimetic drugs of abuse	Cocaine and other sympathomimetic drugs are associated with ICH
Urinalysis and urine culture, as well as a pregnancy test in a woman of childbearing age	
Other routine tests	
Neuroimaging	CT or MRI; consider contrast-enhanced or vascular imaging
ECG	To assess for active coronary ischemia or prior cardiac injury; ECG abnormalities can mark concomitant myocardial injury

Neuroimaging

NCCT and MRI are both used for initial evaluation. For the same reasons mentioned in ischemic stroke chapters, NCCT is more widely used. NCCT is very sensitive for acute hemorrhage and is considered the "gold standard". Gradient echo and T2* susceptibility-weighted MRI are as sensitive as CT for detection of acute hemorrhage and are more sensitive for identification of prior hemorrhage [(1)].

Among patients undergoing NCCT within 3 hours of ICH onset, 28% to 38% have hematoma expansion of greater than one third of the initial hematoma volume on follow-up CT. CT angiography (CTA) and contrast-enhanced CT may identify patients at high risk of ICH expansion based on the presence of contrast within the hematoma, often termed a *spot sign*. A larger number of contrast spots suggests even higher risk of expansion [1].

Underlying vascular abnormalities

Early detection of vascular abnormalities (arteriovenous malformations, vessel-rich tumors, moyamoya, and cerebral vein thrombosis) can both influence clinical management and guide prognosis in ICH patients. Risk factors include age <65 years, female sex, nonsmoker, lobar ICH, intraventricular extension, and absence of a history of hypertension or coagulopathy. Radiological evidence suggestive of vascular abnormalities as causative for ICH can include the presence of subarachnoid hemorrhage, enlarged vessels or calcifications along the margins of the ICH, hyperattenuation within a dural venous sinus or cortical vein along the presumed venous drainage path, unusual hematoma shape, presence of edema out of proportion to the time of presumed ICH, an unusual hemorrhage location, and the presence of other abnormal structures in the brain (like a mass) [1].

MRI, MRA, MRV, and CTA or CT venography (CTV) can identify specific causes of hemorrhage. CTA has been more widely studied and is highly sensitive and specific for detecting vascular abnormalities. DSA may be considered if clinical suspicion is high or noninvasive studies are suggestive of an underlying lesion. MRV or CTV should be performed if hemorrhage location, relative edema volume, or abnormal signal in the cerebral sinuses on routine neuroimaging suggests CVT [1].

Recommendations

1. A baseline severity score should be performed as part of the initial evaluation of patients with ICH *(Class I; Level of Evidence B)*.
2. Rapid neuroimaging with CT or MRI is recommended to distinguish ischemic stroke from ICH *(Class I; Level of Evidence A)*.
3. CTA and contrast-enhanced CT may be considered to help identify patients at risk for hematoma expansion *(Class IIb; Level of Evidence B)*, and CTA, CT venography, contrast-enhanced CT, contrast-enhanced MRI, magnetic resonance angiography and magnetic resonance venography, and catheter angiography can be useful to evaluate for underlying structural lesions including vascular malformations and tumors when there is clinical or radiological suspicion *(Class IIa; Level of Evidence B)*.

Medical treatment for ICH

Hemostasis and Coagulopathy, Antiplatelets, and Deep Vein Thrombosis Prophylaxis

Oral anticoagulant drugs (OACs), antiplatelet agents, acquired or congenital coagulation factor deficiencies, and inherited or acquired qualitative or quantitative platelet abnormalities are risk factors for ICH. OACs cause 12% to 20% of ICH. The newer oral anticoagulants (DOACs) are associated with a lower risk of ICH than vitamin K antagonists (VKAs) [(1)].

Assistance from hematologist is recommended to help reverse hypocoagulability related to coagulation factor deficiency or platelet disorder with replacement of the appropriate factor or platelets. Protamine sulfate 1 mg per 100 U of heparin (maximum dose 50 mg) is used if ICH related to intravenous heparin infusion. Similar dosing can be used in patients who are receiving low-molecular-weight heparin; however, reversal may be incomplete [(1)].

VKA-Related ICH

Fresh frozen plasma (FFP), along with vitamin K, has been the mainstay of treatment. More recently, prothrombin complex concentrates (PCCs), the activated PCC FEIBA (factor VIII inhibitor bypassing activity), and recombinant activated factor VIIa (rFVIIa) have emerged as potential therapies. The goal of reversal is INR < 1.3-1.5 [(1)].

Administration of intravenous vitamin K alone is insufficient for reversal in the first few hours but should be part of all acute VKA reversal strategies in a dose of 5 to 10 mg, usually given slowly via the intravenous route. Onset of action begins by 2 hours and is maximal at ~24 hours if liver function is normal [(1)].

FFP carries a risk of allergic and infectious transfusion reactions, and often requires large volumes for full INR correction. 17% of patients do not achieve INR <1.4 in 24 hours. Shortcomings of FFP have led to interest in alternative agents for VKA reversal [(1)].

PCC can be reconstituted and administered rapidly in a small volume (20–40 mL) and has been processed to inactivate infectious agents. PCCs rapidly normalizes the INR (within minutes). PCCs may increase the risk of thrombotic complications, although this risk appears low [(1)].

rFVIIa can rapidly normalize INR in the setting of VKA-associated ICH. However, it does not replenish all of the vitamin K–dependent factors and may not restore thrombin generation as effectively as PCCs. Thus, rFVIIa is not currently recommended for routine use in warfarin reversal [(1)].

DOACs-Related ICH (Table 13.3)

Experience with reversal of DOACs is limited. The available agents (dabigatran, rivaroxaban, and apixaban) have relatively short half-lives ranging from 5 to 15 hours. Evaluation of the activated partial thromboplastin time and prothrombin time and consultation with a hematologist are reasonable to individualize care [(1)].

Potential reversal strategies using factor eight inhibitor bypassing activity (FEIBA), other PCCs, or rFVIIa might be considered. FFP is of unclear utility, and vitamin K is not useful. It has been suggested that FEIBA or rFVIIa may be better for the direct thrombin inhibitor dabigatran, whereas other PCCs may be better for the factor Xa inhibitors rivaroxaban and apixaban, but these data are preliminary [(1)].

Activated charcoal can be used if the most recent dose of dabigatran, apixaban, or rivaroxaban was taken within couple of hours. Hemodialysis has been noted as an option for dabigatran, but less so for rivaroxaban or apixaban because these are more highly protein bound. Specific antidotes for some DOACs are listed in table 13.3 [(1)].

Antiplatelet–Related ICH

There is no clear correlation of antiplatelet agent use and hematoma expansion. However, platelet dysfunction as measured by platelet function assays may be associated with hematoma expansion. Platelet function monitoring could be helpful in assessing exposure to antiplatelet medications and guiding hemostatic interventions, but this approach has not been fully studied. Two randomized controlled trials are ongoing to evaluate the effectiveness of platelet transfusion in ICH patients taking antiplatelet agents [(1)].

Table 13.3. AHA scientific recommendations for DOACs-related bleed.

<table>
<tr><th colspan="4">DOACs bleeding management protocol (2)</th></tr>
<tr><td colspan="2">General measures</td><td colspan="2">Mechanical compression if possible
Two sites of IV access
Determine timing of last DOAC dose
CBC, BUN, Creatine, liver enzyme
Consider activated charcoal if DOAC ingestion <2hours
Notify on-call hematologist
Refer to chart below for specific measures</td></tr>
<tr><th>DOAC</th><th>Blood tests for DOAC presence or effect</th><th>Special Antidote</th><th>Alternative Treatment Options</th></tr>
<tr><td>Dabigatran</td><td>PTT, TT</td><td>Idarucizumab 5 grams IV (2 infusions of 2.5 grams)</td><td>4 Factor PCC (Kcentra) 50 IU/kg IV
Factor VIIa 90 µg/kg IV every 2 hrs
Tranexamic acid 15-30 mg/kg IV
Hemodialysis</td></tr>
<tr><td>Rivaroxaban</td><td>Anti-Factor Xa</td><td>Andexanet Alfa 400 mg bolus (30 m) then 4 mg/m (up to 120 m)
Double dose if > 10 mg</td><td>4 Factor PCC (Kcentra) 50 IU/kg IV
Factor VIIa 90 µg/kg IV every 2 hrs
Tranexamic acid 15-30 mg/kg IV</td></tr>
<tr><td>Apixaban</td><td>Anti-Factor Xa</td><td>Andexanet Alfa 400 mg bolus (30 m) then 4 mg/min (up to 120 m)
Double dose if > 5 mg</td><td>PCC (Kcentra) 50 IU/kg IV
Factor VIIa 90 µg/kg IV every 2 hrs
Tranexamic acid 15-30 mg/kg IV</td></tr>
<tr><td>Edoxaban</td><td>Anti-Factor Xa</td><td>Unavailable in the US</td><td>PCC (Kcentra) 50 IU/kg IV
Factor VIIa 90 µg/kg IV every 2 hrs
Tranexamic acid 15-30 mg/kg IV</td></tr>
<tr><td colspan="4">TT = thrombin time, PTT = partial thromboplastin time, PCC = prothrombin complex concentrate</td></tr>
</table>

Thrombolytic-Related ICH

After discontinuing thrombolytic agents, it is recommended to use cryoprecipitate (10 units initial dose) if patient is with symptomatic ICH and received a thrombolytic agent in the previous 24 h. (Conditional recommendation, low-quality evidence) [3].

In cases where cryoprecipitate is contraindicated or not available in a timely manner, the use of an antifibrinolytic agent (tranexamic acid 10–15 mg/kg IV over 20 min or e-aminocaproic acid 4–5 g IV) is recommended as an alternative to cryoprecipitate. (Conditional recommendation, very low-quality evidence) [3].

It is recommended to check fibrinogen levels after administration of reversal agents. If the fibrinogen is less than 150 mg/dL, we suggest administration of additional cryoprecipitate. (Conditional recommendation, very low-quality evidence). It is unclear if platelet transfusion is useful and it cannot be recommended at this time [3].

rFVIIa in ICH Not Related to Anticoagulant Agents

Use of rFVIIa was associated with an increased frequency of thromboembolic events. It remains to be determined whether rFVIIa might benefit a particular subset of patients with ICH, but currently its benefits in ICH patients, whether or not they are taking an OAC, remain unproven [1].

Recommendations

1. Patients with a severe coagulation factor deficiency or severe thrombocytopenia should receive appropriate factor replacement therapy or platelets, respectively *(Class I; Level of Evidence* C).

2. Patients with ICH whose INR is elevated because of VKA should have their VKA withheld, receive therapy to replace vitamin K–dependent factors and correct the INR, and receive intravenous vitamin K *(Class I; Level of Evidence C)*. PCCs may have fewer complications and correct the INR more rapidly than FFP and might be considered over FFP *(Class IIb; Level of Evidence B)*. rFVIIa does not replace all clotting factors, and although the INR may be lowered, clotting may not be restored in vivo; therefore, rFVIIa is not recommended for VKA reversal in ICH *(Class III; Level of Evidence C)*.
3. For patients with ICH who are taking dabigatran, rivaroxaban, or apixaban, treatment with FEIBA, other PCCs, or rFVIIa might be considered on an individual basis. Activated charcoal might be used if the most recent dose of dabigatran, apixaban, or rivaroxaban was taken <2 hours earlier. Hemodialysis might be considered for dabigatran *(Class IIb; Level of Evidence C)*.
4. Protamine sulfate may be considered to reverse heparin in patients with acute ICH *(Class IIb; Level of Evidence C)*.
5. The usefulness of platelet transfusions in ICH patients with a history of antiplatelet use is uncertain *(Class IIb; Level of Evidence C)*.
6. Although rFVIIa can limit the extent of hematoma expansion in noncoagulopathic ICH patients, there is an increase in thromboembolic risk with rFVIIa and no clear clinical benefit in unselected patients. Thus, rFVIIa is not recommended *(Class III; Level of Evidence A)*.

Thromboprophylaxis in ICH patients

ICH increases the risk of thromboembolic events especially in women and black. Intermittent pneumatic compression started early (same day of admission) reduces the occurrence of proximal DVT [(1)].

If DVT or PE develop full systemic anticoagulation or placement of an inferior vena cava (IVC) filter may be considered (12% to 15% recurrence rate of PE if not nontreated). Observation alone is not recommended. Only very limited information is available to guide decision making on IVC filter placement versus anticoagulation, as well as the optimal anticoagulation regimen.

Considerations include the post-hemorrhage date on which DVT/PE is diagnosed, documentation of stable hematoma size on neuroimaging, lobar versus deep hematoma location, and the practical ability to remove an IVC filter at a later date. General guidelines for the use of IVC filters in the setting of acute DVT suggest a conventional course of anticoagulant therapy if the risk of bleeding resolves; however, these are not ICH specific [1].

Recommendations:

1. Patients with ICH should have intermittent pneumatic compression for prevention of venous thromboembolism beginning the day of hospital admission *(Class I; Level of Evidence A)*. Graduated compression stockings are not beneficial to reduce DVT or improve outcome *(Class III; Level of Evidence A)*.
2. After documentation of cessation of bleeding, low-dose subcutaneous low-molecular-weight heparin or unfractionated heparin may be considered for prevention of venous thromboembolism in patients with lack of mobility after 1 to 4 days from onset *(Class IIb; Level of Evidence B)*.
3. Systemic anticoagulation or IVC filter placement is probably indicated in ICH patients with symptomatic DVT or PE *(Class IIa; Level of Evidence C)*. The decision between these 2 options should take into account several factors, including time from hemorrhage onset, hematoma stability, cause of hemorrhage, and overall patient condition *(Class IIa; Level of Evidence C)*.

BP and outcome in ICH

Elevated BP is very common in acute ICH because of a variety of factors, including stress, pain, increased ICP, and premorbid acute or persistent elevations in BP. High SBP is associated with greater hematoma expansion, neurological deterioration, and death and dependency after ICH. Compared with ischemic stroke, in which consistent U- or J-shaped associations between SBP nadir of 140 - 150 mm Hg and poor outcome have been shown, only 1 study of ICH has shown a poor outcome at low SBP levels (<140 mm Hg) (1).

Safety of Early Intensive BP-Lowering Treatment

There is no significant reduction in cerebral blood flow within the perihematomal region related to early intensive BP lowering to an SBP target of <140 mm Hg within several hours of ICH. However, there is no clear evidence that BP lowering improves outcome (1).

Efficacy of Early Intensive BP-Lowering Treatment

Overall, current evidence indicates that early intensive BP lowering is safe and feasible and that surviving patients show modestly better functional recovery. It is reasonable to recommend SBP level <140 mm (1).

There are fewer data available pertaining to the safety and effectiveness of such treatment in patients with very high BP (sustained SBP >220 mm Hg) on presentation, large and more severe ICH, and those requiring surgical decompression. Because the speed and degree of BP reduction will vary according to the agent and method of delivery (bolus versus infusion) and clinical features, the agent of choice should take into account the practicability, pharmacological profile, potential side effects, and cost (1).

Recommendations

1. For ICH patients presenting with SBP between 150 and 220 mmHg and without contraindication to acute BP treatment, acute lowering of SBP to 140 mmHg is safe *(Class I; Level of Evidence A)* and can be effective for improving functional outcome *(Class IIa; Level of Evidence B)*.

2. For ICH patients presenting with SBP >220 mmHg, it may be reasonable to consider aggressive reduction of BP with a continuous intravenous infusion and frequent BP monitoring *(Class IIb; Level of Evidence C)*.

Inpatient management and prevention of secondary brain injury

General Monitoring

Patients with ICH are frequently medically and neurologically unstable, particularly within the first few days after onset. Care of ICH patients in a dedicated neuroscience intensive care unit (NICU) is associated with a lower mortality rate. Frequent vital sign checks, neurological assessments, and continuous cardiopulmonary monitoring including a cycled automated BP cuff, electrocardiographic telemetry, and pulse oximetry probe should be standard. Continuous intra-arterial BP monitoring should be considered in patients receiving intravenous vasoactive medications [(1)].

Nursing Care

The specific nursing care required for ICH patients in intensive care units may include 1) surveillance and monitoring of ICP, cerebral perfusion pressure (CPP), and hemodynamic function; 2) titration and implementation of protocols for management of ICP, BP, mechanical ventilation, fever, and serum glucose; and 3) prevention of complications of immobility through positioning, airway maintenance, and mobilization within physiological tolerance. The consensus document from the Brain Attack Coalition on comprehensive stroke centers delineates these as specific areas of monitoring and complication prevention in which nurses should be trained. This document also recommends that nurses be trained in detailed assessment of neurological function, including standardized scales such as the NIHSS, GCS, and the Glasgow Outcome Scale [1].

Recommendation

1. Initial monitoring and management of ICH patients should take place in an intensive care unit or dedicated stroke unit with physician and nursing neuroscience acute care expertise *(Class I; Level of Evidence B)*.

Glucose management

High blood glucose on admission predicts an increased risk of mortality and poor outcome in patients with ICH, independent of the presence of diabetes mellitus. The optimal management of hyperglycemia in ICH and the target glucose level remains to be clarified. Hypoglycemia should be avoided [1].

Recommendation

1. Glucose should be monitored. Both hyperglycemia and hypoglycemia should be avoided *(Class I; Level of Evidence C)*.

Temperature management

Fever is common after ICH, especially with IVH. In patients surviving the first 72 hours after hospital admission, the duration of fever is related to outcome and appears to be an independent prognostic factor in these patients. Fever may also be associated with hematoma growth, although a cause-effect relationship is unclear. Although these data provide a rationale for treatment of fever in ICH patients, maintenance of normothermia has not been clearly demonstrated as beneficial to outcome. Therapeutic cooling may reduce perihematomal edema. However, treatment with mild hypothermia should be considered investigational in ICH at this time [1].

Recommendation

1. Treatment of fever after ICH may be reasonable *(Class IIb; Level of Evidence C)*.

Seizures and antiseizure drugs

Early seizure (within 1 week) after ICH rate is 16%. Cortical ICH is the most important risk factor for early seizures. There is no clear association between clinical seizures and neurological outcome or mortality. Prophylactic antiseizure drugs significantly reduced the number of clinical seizures after lobar ICH [1].

Studies of continuous electroencephalography (EEG) report electrographic seizures in 28% to 31% of ICH patients, despite most having received prophylactic antiseizure medications. The clinical impact of subclinical seizures detected on EEG is unclear [1].

Clinical seizures or electrographic seizures in patients with a change in mental status should be treated with antiseizure drugs. Continuous EEG monitoring should be considered in ICH patients with depressed mental status that is disproportionate to the degree of brain injury [1].

Epilepsy occurs in up to 10% of young patients (18–50 years) with ICH; the risk of poststroke epilepsy may be less in older patients. Risk factors for epilepsy include stroke severity, cortical location of the hematoma, and delayed initial seizures. There are no data to suggest that early use of antiseizure drugs will prevent lesion-related epilepsy [(1)].

Recommendations

1. Clinical seizures should be treated with antiseizure drugs *(Class I; Level of Evidence A)*.
2. Patients with a change in mental status who are found to have electrographic seizures on EEG should be treated with antiseizure drugs *(Class I; Level of Evidence C)*.
3. Continuous EEG monitoring is probably indicated in ICH patients with depressed mental status that is out of proportion to the degree of brain injury *(Class IIa; Level of Evidence C)*.
4. Prophylactic antiseizure medication is not recommended *(Class III; Level of Evidence B)*.

Management of medical complications

The most common medical complications are pneumonia (5.6%), aspiration (2.6%), respiratory failure/distress (2%), PE (1.3%), and sepsis (1.7%). Approximately 50% of deaths after stroke are attributed to medical complications, usually after 7 days of hospitalization. Stroke patients who experience medical complications while in the hospital have increased mortality up to 4 years after the initial event [(1)].

Dysphagia and aspiration are major risk factors for the development of pneumonia.

Serious cardiac events and cardiac death after stroke may be caused by acute myocardial infarction (MI), heart failure, ventricular arrhythmias including ventricular tachycardia/fibrillation, and cardiac arrest. For ICH patients, an elevated troponin level >0.4 ng/mL was found in 15% within 24 hours of admission and was associated with increased in-hospital mortality. Heart failure can occur as the result of myocardial ischemia, infarction, stress-induced cardiomyopathy, or uncontrolled hypertension in the setting of acute ICH [(1)].

Neurogenic pulmonary edema is an increase in interstitial and alveolar fluid in the setting of an acute central nervous system injury well documented in subarachnoid hemorrhage but prevalent in ICH as well. Resolution usually occurs within several days. Intubation with mechanical ventilator support is often required for airway protection and maximum oxygen delivery [(1)].

Recommendations

1. A formal screening procedure for dysphagia should be performed in all patients before the initiation of oral intake to reduce the risk of pneumonia *(Class I; Level of Evidence B)*.
2. Systematic screening for myocardial ischemia or infarction with electrocardiogram and cardiac enzyme testing after ICH is reasonable *(Class IIa; Level of Evidence C)*.

▪ Procedures/surgery

ICP Monitoring and Treatment

Increased ICP is more common in younger patients and those with supratentorial ICH. Hydrocephalus is associated with worsened outcome in ICH [(1)].

Rising ICP and declining CPP are associated with mortality. ICP monitoring and subsequent treatment might be considered in ICH patients with a GCS score of ≤ 8 that is presumed related to hematoma mass effect, those with clinical evidence of transtentorial herniation, or those with significant IVH or hydrocephalus. Thus, it is recommended to place an ICP monitor in patients with a GCS score of 3 to 8 and to maintain an ICP <20 mm Hg and a CPP of 50 to 70 mm Hg, depending on the status of cerebral autoregulation (1).

Methods of treating elevated ICP are also borrowed from traumatic brain injury guidelines as well. Basic principles include: 1) elevation of the head of the bed to 30°, 2) the use of mild sedation, 3) avoidance of collar-endotracheal tube ties that might constrict cervical veins. Mannitol or hypertonic saline may be used to treat acute ICP elevations, and hypertonic saline may be more effective. In patients with CSF outflow obstruction caused by hydrocephalus or a trapped ventricle, CSF drainage should be considered. Hematoma evacuation (HE) and decompressive craniectomy (DC) are options for treating elevated ICP and are discussed in the section on Surgical Treatment of ICH. Salvage therapies might include barbiturate coma or mild hypothermia. Corticosteroids should not be used, because they are not effective in ICH and increase complications (1).

Recommendations

1. Ventricular drainage as treatment for hydrocephalus is reasonable, especially in patients with decreased level of consciousness *(Class IIa; Level of Evidence B)*.
2. Patients with a GCS score of ≤8, those with clinical evidence of transtentorial herniation, or those with significant IVH or hydrocephalus might be considered for ICP monitoring and treatment. A CPP of 50 to 70 mmHg may be reasonable to maintain depending on the status of cerebral autoregulation *(Class IIb; Level of Evidence C)*.
3. Corticosteroids should not be administered for treatment of elevated ICP in ICH *(Class III; Level of Evidence B)*.

▪ Intraventricular hemorrhage (IVH)

IVH occurs in ~ 45% of patients with spontaneous ICH and is associated with poor outcome and death (20% without IVH, 51% with IVH). Ventricular catheter (VC) should theoretically aid in drainage of blood and CSF from the ventricles; however, VC use alone may be ineffective because of difficulty maintaining catheter patency and the slow removal of intraventricular blood. Thus, there has been recent interest in the use of thrombolytic agents as adjuncts to VC use in the setting of IVH [(1)].

Intraventricular thrombolytic infusion through VC reduces mortality from 30% to 10%. Studies with rtPA have used various dose regimens ranging from 1 to 4 mg every 8 to 12 hours [(1)].

There are recent reports of alternative procedures for IVH, such as endoscopic surgical evacuation and ventriculostomy. Endoscopic removal of IVH is associated with 17% need for permanent CSF diversion compared with 50% of patients treated with VC alone. Other reported management strategies for IVH include early ventriculoperitoneal shunting, endoscopic third ventriculostomy, or lumbar drainage. Patient managed with VC plus lumbar drainage had a longer median duration of external CSF drainage but were significantly less likely to require permanent CSF diversion [(1)].

Recommendations

1. Although intraventricular administration of rtPA in IVH appears to have a fairly low complication rate, the efficacy and safety of this treatment are uncertain *(Class IIb; Level of Evidence B)*.
2. The efficacy of endoscopic treatment of IVH is uncertain *(Class IIb; Level of Evidence B)*.

Surgical treatment of ICH (clot removal)

The role of surgery for most patients with spontaneous ICH remains controversial. The theoretical rationale for hematoma evacuation (HE) revolves around the concepts of preventing herniation, reducing ICP, and decreasing the pathophysiological impact of the hematoma on surrounding tissue by decreasing mass effect or the cellular toxicity of blood products [(1)].

Craniotomy for Supratentorial ICH

There is no overall statistically significant improvement in mortality or functional outcome with craniotomy even when done early. However, patient with lobar hemorrhages within 1 cm of the cortical surface might benefit from surgery. There is likely no benefit from craniotomy in patients who presented with coma (GCS score ≤8) [(1)].

Craniotomy for Posterior Fossa ICH

Because of the narrow confines of the posterior fossa, deterioration can occur quickly in cerebellar hemorrhage caused by obstructive hydrocephalus or local mass effect on the brainstem.

There is significant benefit from surgical decompression in cerebellar hemorrhages >3 cm in diameter or patients in whom cerebellar hemorrhage is associated with brainstem compression or hydrocephalus.

Attempting to control ICP via means other than hematoma evacuation, such as VC insertion alone, is considered insufficient, is not recommended, and may actually be harmful, particularly in patients with compressed cisterns.

In contrast to cerebellar hemorrhage, evacuation of brainstem hemorrhages may be harmful in many cases. Given the broad lack of clinical equipoise for surgical evacuation of cerebellar hemorrhages, especially those >3 cm in diameter occurring in potentially salvageable patients, it is unlikely that a randomized trial could be conducted to compare surgery versus conservative treatment [(1)].

Decompressive Craniectomy (DC) for ICH

The potential of DC to improve outcomes for patients with ICH has not been well studied. A systematic review of studies in which DC was performed in the setting of spontaneous ICH suggested that DC with hematoma evacuation might be safe and might improve outcomes [(1)].

Minimally Invasive Surgical Evacuation (MISE) of ICH

Several recent randomized studies have compared MISE to standard craniotomies and suggested better outcomes with less invasive approaches. The Minimally Invasive Surgery Plus Recombinant Tissue-Type Plasminogen Activator for ICH Evacuation Trial II (MISTIE II) demonstrated a significant reduction in perihematomal edema in the hematoma evacuation group with a trend toward improved outcomes [(1)].

Timing of Surgery

Timing of surgery for ICH remains controversial (4 to 96 hours). However, there is trend toward better outcome for patients operated on before 21 hours from ictus and especially within 8 hours of hemorrhage. Ultra-early craniotomy (within 4 hours from ictus) was associated with an increased risk of rebleeding in a study that involved 24 patients [(1)].

Recommendations

1. Patients with cerebellar hemorrhage who are deteriorating neurologically or who have brainstem compression and/or

hydrocephalus from ventricular obstruction should undergo surgical removal of the hemorrhage as soon as possible *(Class I; Level of Evidence B)*. Initial treatment of these patients with ventricular drainage rather than surgical evacuation is not recommended *(Class III; Level of Evidence C)*.

2. For most patients with supratentorial ICH, the usefulness of surgery is not well established *(Class IIb; Level of Evidence A)*. Specific exceptions and potential subgroup considerations are outlined below in recommendations 3 through 6.
3. A policy of early hematoma evacuation is not clearly beneficial compared with hematoma evacuation when patients deteriorate *(Class IIb; Level of Evidence A)*.
4. Supratentorial hematoma evacuation in deteriorating patients might be considered as a life-saving measure *(Class IIb; Level of Evidence C)*.
5. DC with or without hematoma evacuation might reduce mortality for patients with supratentorial ICH who are in a coma, have large hematomas with significant midline shift, or have elevated ICP refractory to medical management *(Class IIb; Level of Evidence C)*.
6. The effectiveness of minimally invasive clot evacuation with stereotactic or endoscopic aspiration with or without thrombolytic usage is uncertain *(Class IIb; Level of Evidence B)*.

Outcome prediction and withdrawal of technological support

As discussed in chapter 2, GCS or NIHSS, age, hematoma volume and location, and the presence and amount of IVH can predict outcome. However, most patients who die of ICH do so during the initial acute hospitalization, and these deaths usually occur in the setting of withdrawal of support because of presumed poor prognosis. The decision to limit care early after ICH may therefore result in self-fulfilling prophecies of poor outcome, and studies show that current outcome prediction models are overly pessimistic because of the failure to account for these care limitations [(1)].

Recommendation

1. Aggressive care early after ICH onset and postponement of new DNAR orders until at least the second full day of hospitalization is probably recommended *(Class IIa; Level of Evidence B)*.
2. Patients with preexisting DNAR orders are not included in this recommendation. Current prognostic models for individual patients early after ICH are biased by failure to account for the influence of withdrawal of support and early DNAR orders. DNAR status should not limit appropriate medical and surgical interventions unless otherwise explicitly indicated *(Class III; Level of Evidence C)*.

Prevention of recurrent ICH

Patients with ICH are at high risk of a recurrent event and of other major vascular disease. The cumulative risk of ICH recurrence is 1% to 5% per year. Although the risk of ICH recurrence is highest in the first year after the initial event, the ongoing risk extends for years, particularly in patients with lobar ICH [(1)].

Risk Factors

Hypertension, older age, and location of the initial hemorrhage (lobar > deep) are important risk factors for ICH recurrence. Increased risk in the elderly is due to cerebral amyloid angiopathy (CAA) and increased use of antithrombotic medications with accumulating comorbidities.

CAA is a recognized risk factor for recurrent ICH, particularly in lobar locations. Carriers of the apolipoprotein E $\varepsilon 2$ or $\varepsilon 4$ alleles, patients with previous ICH before the presenting ICH, and patients with a greater number of microbleeds (particularly microbleeds in lobar brain locations) on gradient echo MRI appear to be at higher risk for ICH recurrence.

In whites, most of the initial and recurrent hemorrhages tend to be lobar, whereas deep hemorrhages (both initial and recurrent) are more common in Asians.

A history of ischemic stroke, particularly of the small-vessel "lacunar" type, which shares a common pathogenesis with ICH, might also be a predictor of ICH recurrence [(1)].

Recommendations

1. When stratifying a patient's risk for recurrent ICH may affect management decisions, it is reasonable to consider the following risk factors for ICH recurrence: (1) lobar location of the initial ICH; (2) older age; (3) presence and number of microbleeds on gradient echo MRI; (4) ongoing anticoagulation; and (5) presence of apolipoprotein E ε2 or ε4 alleles *(Class IIa; Level of Evidence B)*.

▪ BP Management

Among ICH risk factors, only BP and the use of antithrombotic agents are modifiable. The optimal timing for initiating BP lowering after ICH to prevent recurrence is unknown. Rapid reduction of SBP to <140 mm Hg within a few hours is safe, which indicates that such treatment can be safely initiated as soon as possible after ICH onset. ICH patients should have their BP lowered to or beyond the targets currently recommended in other high-risk groups (<130 mm Hg systolic and 80 mm Hg diastolic in the presence of diabetes mellitus, heart failure, or chronic kidney disease) [(1)].

Other factors, such as BP variability, the presence of obstructive sleep apnea, obesity, and other lifestyle modifications, should also be considered despite the lack of systematic data regarding their effect on ICH recurrence. Frequent alcohol use (>2 drinks per day) and illicit drug use have been linked to elevated

BP and ICH and should be avoided in ICH patients. Tobacco use is also associated with increased ICH risk and should be discontinued [(1)].

Recommendations

1. BP should be controlled in all ICH patients *(Class I; Level of Evidence A)*. **(Revised from the previous guideline)** Measures to control BP should begin immediately after ICH onset *(Class I; Level of Evidence A)*. A long-term goal of BP <130 mmHg systolic and 80 mmHg diastolic is reasonable *(Class IIa; Level of Evidence B)*.

Management of antithrombotic drugs

The rising use of anticoagulant agents in an aging population is associated with increased risk of ICH and its recurrence. History of ICH is not absolute contraindication for restarting anticoagulant [(1)].

The optimal timing for resumption of anticoagulation after ICH, if necessary, is uncertain, and no randomized trial data are available to guide the decision [(1)].

In practice, the timing often depends on the indication for anticoagulation. In patients with prosthetic heart valves, early resumption of anticoagulation may be necessary because of the high risk of embolism. Although there are conflicting reports regarding the risk of ICH recurrence with antiplatelet use, particularly in patients with lobar ICH, antiplatelet monotherapy or percutaneous left atrial appendage closure may be safer alternatives to warfarin in some patients with atrial fibrillation. Antiplatelet agents do not appear to dramatically increase the risk of hematoma expansion and therefore appear to be generally safe for use after ICH, including ICH caused by CAA [(1)].

Although dabigatran, rivaroxaban, and apixaban are reported to convey a lower risk of ICH than warfarin in atrial fibrillation patients, their usefulness as alternatives to warfarin after ICH remains to be determined (1).

Recommendations

1. Lifestyle modifications, including avoidance of alcohol use greater than 2 drinks per day, tobacco use, and illicit drug use, as well as treatment of obstructive sleep apnea, are probably beneficial *(Class IIa; Level of Evidence B)*.
2. Avoidance of long-term anticoagulation with warfarin as a treatment for nonvalvular atrial fibrillation is probably recommended after warfarin-associated spontaneous lobar ICH because of the relatively high risk of recurrence *(Class IIa; Level of Evidence B)*.
3. Anticoagulation after nonlobar ICH and antiplatelet monotherapy after any ICH might be considered, particularly when there are strong indications for these agents *(Class IIb; Level of Evidence B)*.
4. The optimal timing to resume oral anticoagulation after anticoagulant-related ICH is uncertain. Avoidance of oral anticoagulation for at least 4 weeks, in patients without mechanical heart valves, might decrease the risk of ICH recurrence *(Class IIb; Level of Evidence B)*. If indicated, aspirin monotherapy can probably be restarted in the days after ICH, although the optimal timing is uncertain *(Class IIa; Level of Evidence B)*.
5. The usefulness of dabigatran, rivaroxaban, or apixaban in patients with atrial fibrillation and past ICH to decrease the risk of recurrence is uncertain *(Class IIb; Level of Evidence C)*.
6. There are insufficient data to recommend restrictions on the use of statins in ICH patients *(Class IIb; Level of Evidence C)*.

Cholesterol Lowering Agents

There are conflicting reports regarding the use of statins in patients with ICH. In the Stroke Prevention With Aggressive Reduction in Cholesterol Levels (SPARCL) study, the benefit of high-dose atorvastatin in reducing recurrent ischemic stroke was offset in part by an increased risk of ICH. A Markov analysis evaluating the risks and benefits of statin therapy in patients with prior ICH concluded that if statin use does increase the risk of ICH, avoidance of statins should be considered in patients with ICH, particularly those with lobar ICH. Concordant with these conclusions, statin use and age were independently associated with the presence and number of microbleeds, especially in cortical locations, in ICH patients. In contrast, continued statin use after ICH was associated with early neurological improvement and reduced 6-month mortality in a small retrospective study. There are no data on whether the reported propensity for ICH with statin use is dose dependent [(1)].

It remains unclear whether statins should be continued or discontinued in ICH patients [(1)].

Rehabilitation and recovery

Even so, there is growing evidence that patients with ICH make slightly greater and faster gains in recovery than patients with ischemic stroke. In general, recovery is more rapid in the first few weeks but may continue for many months after ICH, with approximately half of all survivors remaining dependent on others for activities of daily living. Cognition, mood, motivation, and social support all influence recovery, and it is difficult to separate intrinsic from adaptive recovery.

A simple prognostic score that uses 1) age, 2) ICH volume and location, 3) level of consciousness at admission, and 4) pre-ICH cognitive impairment has been shown to predict independence at 90 days. Such scores are useful across all patients, but prognostic imaging techniques may also be useful with lesions in specific functional areas. Given that ICH is often located in lobar regions and complicated by intraventricular extension, some patients with specific cognitive deficits or delayed recovery that is disproportionate to the size of the lesion may require specialized therapy in rehabilitation [1].

The success of rehabilitation depends on caregiver training and support; however, the likely configuration of services in any region will depend on available resources and funding options.

A key portion of rehabilitation should include education for the patient and caregiver regarding secondary stroke prevention and means to achieve rehabilitation goals. Rehabilitation programs should consider lifestyle changes, depression, and caregiver burden as important issues to address with the patient and caregivers [1].

Recommendations

1. Given the potentially serious nature and complex pattern of evolving disability and the increasing evidence for efficacy, it is recommended that all patients with ICH have access to multidisciplinary rehabilitation *(Class I; Level of Evidence A)*.
2. Where possible, rehabilitation can be beneficial when begun as early as possible and continued in the community as part of a well-coordinated ("seamless") program of accelerated hospital discharge and home-based resettlement to promote ongoing recovery *(Class IIa; Level of Evidence B)*.

References

1. *Guidelines for the Management of Spontaneous Intracerebral Hemorrhage A Guideline for Healthcare Professionals From the American Heart Association/American Stroke Association.* J. Claude HemphillIII, Steven M. Greenberg , Craig S. Anderson. s.l. : Stroke, 2015, Vol. 46.
2. *Management of Patients on Non–Vitamin K Antagonist Oral Anticoagulants in the Acute Care and Periprocedural SettingA Scientific Statement From the American Heart Association.* Amish N. Raval, MD, FAHA, ChairJoaquin E. Cigarroa, MDMina K. Chung, MD, FAHA. s.l. : Circulation, 2017, Vol. 135.
3. *Guideline for Reversal of Antithrombotics in Intracranial Hemorrhage.* Jennifer A. Frontera, John J. Lewin III, Alejandro A. Rabinstein. 6, s.l. : Neuro Critical Care, 2016, Vol. 24.

14

Management of Aneurysmal Subarachnoid Hemorrhage (aSAH)

aSAH is a significant cause of morbidity and mortality. 25% of patients die, and 50% of survivors remain with persistent neurological deficit. However, early aneurysm repair, together with aggressive management of complications such as hydrocephalus and delayed cerebral ischemia (DCI), improves functional outcomes [(1)]. Please refer to table 10.2 for strength and level of evidence while reading the following guidelines and recommendations.

▪ Incidence and prevalence of aSAH

Annual incidence of aSAH ranges from 2.0 cases per 100,000 population in China to 22.5 cases per 100,000 in Finland. aSAH is relatively uncommon in children; incidence rates increase as children get older, with incidence ranging from 0.18 to 2.0 per 100 000. The majority of studies also indicate a higher incidence of aSAH in women than in men. Blacks and Hispanics have a higher incidence of aSAH than white Americans [1].

Risk factors for and prevention of aSAH

There are modifiable and non-modifiable risk factors for forming cerebral aneurysm (discussed in chapter 2). In addition to these factors, there are several risk factors for aneurysm rupture such as female sex, symptomatic aneurysm, larger size, posterior communicating artery or vertebrobasilar location, previous aSAH, a history of familial aneurysms (at least 1 first-degree family member with an intracranial aneurysm, and especially if >2 first- degree relatives are affected) and family history of aSAH, and certain genetic syndromes, such as autosomal dominant polycystic kidney disease and type IV Ehlers-Danlos syndrome [1]. Also, many other risk factors are included in PHASES score discussed in chapter 2 (Table 2.1).

Given such uncertainties, younger age, longer life expectancy, and higher rate of rupture all make treatment of unruptured aneurysms more likely to be cost-effective and reduce morbidity and mortality [1].

Recommendations

1. Treatment of high blood pressure with antihypertensive medication is recommended to prevent ischemic stroke, intracerebral hemorrhage, and cardiac, renal, and other end-organ injury *(Class I; Level of Evidence A).*
2. Hypertension should be treated, and such treatment may reduce the risk of aSAH *(Class I; Level of Evidence B).*
3. Tobacco use and alcohol misuse should be avoided to reduce the risk of aSAH *(Class I; Level of Evidence B).*

4. In addition to the size and location of the aneurysm and the patient's age and health status, it might be reasonable to consider morphological and hemodynamic characteristics of the aneurysm when discussing the risk of aneurysm rupture *(Class IIb; Level of Evidence B).*
5. Consumption of a diet rich in vegetables may lower the risk of aSAH *(Class IIb; Level of Evidence B).*
6. It may be reasonable to offer noninvasive screening to patients with familial (at least 1 first-degree relative) aSAH and/or a history of aSAH to evaluate for de novo aneurysms or late regrowth of a treated aneurysm, but the risks and benefits of this screening require further study *(Class IIb; Level of Evidence B).*
7. After any aneurysm repair, immediate cerebrovascular imaging is generally recommended to identify remnants or recurrence of the aneurysm that may require treatment *(Class I; Level of Evidence B).*

Natural history and outcome of aSAH

Mortality from aSAH has declined in industrialized nations over the past 25 years. In the US, there is a decrease of 1% per year from 1979 to 1994. However, global cognitive impairment is still present in 20% of aSAH patients and is associated with poorer functional recovery and lower quality of life. Cognitive deficits and functional decline are often compounded by mood disorders (anxiety, depression), fatigue, and sleep disturbances. The severity of clinical presentation and rebleeding are the strongest prognostic indicator of poor cognition in aSAH. Other factors predictive of poor prognosis include older age, preexisting severe medical illness, global cerebral edema on computed tomography (CT) scan, intraventricular and intracerebral hemorrhage, symptomatic vasospasm, delayed cerebral infarction (especially if multiple), hyperglycemia, fever, anemia, and other systemic complications such as pneumonia and sepsis. Treatment in high-volume centers with availability of neurosurgical and endovascular services may be associated with better outcomes [1].

Recommendations

1. The initial clinical severity of aSAH should be determined rapidly by use of simple validated scales (eg, Hunt and Hess, World Federation of Neurological Surgeons), because it is the most useful indicator of outcome after aSAH *(Class I; Level of Evidence B).*
2. The risk of early aneurysm rebleeding is high, and rebleeding is associated with very poor outcomes. Therefore, urgent evaluation and treatment of patients with suspected aSAH is recommended *(Class I; Level of Evidence B).*
3. After discharge, it is reasonable to refer patients with aSAH for a comprehensive evaluation, including cognitive, behavioral, and psychosocial assessments *(Class IIa; Level of Evidence B).*

Clinical manifestations and diagnosis of aSAH

The hallmark (80% of cases) of aSAH is "the worst headache of my life", which is extremely sudden with immediate maximal intensity (thunderclap headache). 10-43 % of patients develop warning or sentinel headache that precedes the worst headache. aSAH can occur during physical exertion or stress; however, the highest incidence of rupture occurred while patients were engaged in their daily routines. Other findings are nausea/ vomiting, stiff neck, photophobia, brief loss of consciousness, or focal neurological deficits (including cranial nerve palsies) [1].

Misdiagnosis is not uncommon and is associated with 4-fold increase of death or disability at 1 year in patients with minimal or no neurological deficit at the initial visit. The most common diagnostic error is failure to obtain a NCCT [1].

Seizures may occur in up to 20% of patients after aSAH, most commonly in the first 24 hours and more commonly in aSAH associated with intracerebral hemorrhage, hypertension, and middle cerebral and anterior communicating artery aneurysms [(1)].

Imaging

NCCT is the cornerstone of diagnosis of aSAH. The sensitivity of CT in the first 3 days after aSAH is close to 100%, after which it decreases moderately during the next few days. After 5 to 7 days, the rate of negative CT increases sharply, and lumbar puncture is often required to show xanthochromia. However, advances in MRI of the brain, particularly the use of FLAIR, proton density (PD), DWI, and gradient echo sequences (GRE), can often allow the diagnosis of aSAH to be made when a head CT scan is negative and there is clinical suspicion of aSAH, possibly avoiding the need for lumbar puncture [(1)].

CTA is the first line vascular non-invasive imaging modality to detect aneurysm; however, aneurysms < 3 mm in size cannot be reliably demonstrated on CTA [(1)].

DSA is still widely used in the investigation of aSAH and the characterization of ruptured cerebral aneurysms. The combination of 3- and 2-dimensional DSA usually provides the best morphological depiction of aneurysm anatomy with high spatial resolution, and it is, of course, always used in preparation for endovascular therapy [(1)].

Recommendations

1. aSAH is a medical emergency that is frequently misdiagnosed. A high level of suspicion for aSAH should exist in patients with acute onset of severe headache *(Class I; Level of Evidence B)*.

2. Acute diagnostic workup should include noncontrast head CT, which, if nondiagnostic, should be followed by lumbar puncture *(Class I; Level of Evidence B).*
3. CTA may be considered in the workup of aSAH. If an aneurysm is detected by CTA, this study may help guide the decision for type of aneurysm repair, but if CTA is inconclusive, DSA is still recommended (except possibly in the instance of classic perimesencephalic aSAH) *(Class IIb; Level of Evidence C).*
4. Magnetic resonance imaging (FLAIR, PD, DWI, and GRE sequences) may be reasonable for the diagnosis of aSAH in patients with a nondiagnostic CT scan, although a negative result does not obviate the need for cerebrospinal fluid analysis *(Class IIb; Level of Evidence C).*
5. DSA with 3-dimensional rotational angiography is indicated for detection of aneurysm in patients with aSAH (except when the aneurysm was previously diagnosed by a noninvasive angiogram) and for planning treatment (to determine whether an aneurysm is amenable to coiling or to expedite microsurgery) *(Class I; Level of Evidence B).*

Medical measures to prevent rebleeding after aSAH

Aneurysm rebleeding is associated with very high mortality and poor prognosis for functional recovery in survivors. The risk of rebleeding is maximal in the first 2 to 12 hours (50% of cases within 6 hours), with reported rates of occurrence between 4% and 13.6% within the first 24 hours. Early rebleeding is associated with worse outcome than later rebleeding [1].

Factors associated with aneurysm rebleeding include longer time to aneurysm treatment, worse neurological status on admission, initial loss of consciousness, previous sentinel headaches, larger aneurysm size, and possibly systolic blood pressure > 160 mm Hg. Early treatment of the ruptured aneurysm can reduce the risk of rebleeding [(1)].

There is general agreement that acute hypertension should be controlled after aSAH and until aneurysm obliteration, but parameters for blood pressure control have not been defined [(1)]. The author recommends keeping SBP < 140 till aneurysm is obliterated (goals can be adjusted based on ICP value).

Short-term use of aminocaproic acid to prevent rebleeding decreases incidence in rebleeding without increasing the risk of DCI. Neither aminocaproic acid nor tranexamic acid is approved by the US Food and Drug Administration for prevention of aneurysm rebleeding [(1)].

Recommendations

1. Between the time of aSAH symptom onset and aneurysm obliteration, blood pressure should be controlled with a titratable agent to balance the risk of stroke, hypertension-related rebleeding, and maintenance of cerebral perfusion pressure *(Class I; Level of Evidence B).*
2. The magnitude of blood pressure control to reduce the risk of rebleeding has not been established, but a decrease in systolic blood pressure to <160 mm Hg is reasonable *(Class IIa; Level of Evidence C).*
3. For patients with an unavoidable delay in obliteration of aneurysm, a significant risk of rebleeding, and no compelling medical contraindications, short- term (<72 hours) therapy with tranexamic acid or aminocaproic acid is reasonable to reduce the risk of early aneurysm rebleeding *(Class IIa; Level of Evidence B).*

Surgical and endovascular treatment of ruptured aneurysms

Microsurgical clipping was the primary modality of treatment before 1991, when Guglielmi invented the endovascular approach using electrolytically detachable coils [1]. More details about surgical clipping techniques used to treat ruptured and unruptured aneurysms are discussed in chapter 15.

There have been multiple efforts to identify subgroups of patients who might be best treated with endovascular or microsurgical techniques. However, there are no clear-cut guidelines to choose one treatment over the other.

Endovascular aneurysm treatment is now the most commonly used technique to obliterate cerebral aneurysms; however, there are some guiding principles.

Middle cerebral artery aneurysms are easily amenable to surgical treatment (older patients are ideal candidates for coiling). Patient with associated ICH > 50 mL would benefit (despite higher unfavorable outcome) from hematoma evacuation within 3.5 hours and microsurgery can be done at the same time through same craniotomy site.

On the other hand, patients presenting during the vasospasm period, especially those with confirmed vasospasm are more suited to endovascular techniques. Also, patients presenting with poor clinical grade benefit more from endovascular coiling, especially if they are elderly. Endovascular treatment is especially safer in posterior circulation aneurysms [1].

There are many endovascular options to treat cerebral aneurysm (micro coil embolization, balloon assist coil embolization, stent assist coil embolization, flow diverters); however, in ruptured aneurysms, the use of stent assist coil embolization and flow diverter requires dual antiplatelet therapy that is considered risky in patients with SAH especially with ventricular drain. However, there are some ruptured aneurysms that are not amenable to surgical or traditional endovascular treatment such as blister aneurysm where flow diverter is the only option. The author performed many cases of flow diverter implantation for ruptured blister aneurysm and published some of the cases in SVIN meeting [2]. More details about endovascular techniques used to treat ruptured and unruptured aneurysms are discussed in chapter 15.

Recommendations

1. Surgical clipping or endovascular coiling of the ruptured aneurysm should be performed as early as feasible in the majority of patients to reduce the rate of rebleeding after aSAH *(Class I; Level of Evidence B).*
2. Complete obliteration of the aneurysm is recommended whenever possible *(Class I; Level of Evidence B).*
3. Determination of aneurysm treatment, as judged by both experienced cerebrovascular surgeons and endovascular specialists, should be a multidisciplinary decision based on characteristics of the patient and the aneurysm *(Class I; Level of Evidence C).*
4. For patients with ruptured aneurysms judged to be technically amenable to both endovascular coiling and neurosurgical clipping, endovascular coiling should be considered *(Class I; Level of Evidence B).*
5. In the absence of a compelling contraindication, patients who undergo coiling or clipping of a ruptured aneurysm should have delayed follow-up vascular imaging (timing and modality to be individualized), and strong consideration should be given to retreatment, either by repeat coiling or microsurgical clipping, if there is a clinically significant (eg, growing) remnant *(Class I; Level of Evidence B).*
6. Microsurgical clipping may receive increased consideration in patients presenting with large (>50 mL) intraparenchymal hematomas and middle cerebral artery aneurysms. Endovascular coiling may receive increased consideration in the elderly (>70 years of age), in those presenting with poor-grade (World Federation of Neurological Surgeons classification IV/V) aSAH, and in those with aneurysms of the basilar apex *(Class IIb; Level of Evidence C).*
7. Stenting of a ruptured aneurysm is associated with increased morbidity and mortality, and should only be considered when less risky options have been excluded *(Class III; Level of Evidence C).*

▪ Hospital characteristics and systems of care

Institutions that use endovascular coil embolization more frequently had lower in-hospital mortality rates, a 9% reduction in risk for every 10% of cases treated. In addition, there was a 16% reduction in risk of in-hospital death at institutions that used interventional therapies such as balloon angioplasty to treat arterial vasospasm. Therefore, hospital treatment volumes and availability of both endovascular and neurological intensive care services at hospitals are important determinants of improved outcomes in aSAH [(1)].

Recommendations

1. Low-volume hospitals (eg, <10 aSAH cases per year) should consider early transfer of patients with aSAH to high-volume centers (eg, >35 aSAH cases per year) with experienced cerebrovascular surgeons, endovascular specialists, and multidisciplinary neuro-intensive care services *(Class I; Level of Evidence B).*
2. Annual monitoring of complication rates for surgical and interventional procedures is reasonable *(Class IIa; Level of Evidence* C).
3. A hospital credentialing process to ensure that proper training standards have been met by individual physicians treating brain aneurysms is reasonable *(Class IIa; Level of Evidence C).*

▪ Anesthetic management during surgical and endovascular treatment

The general goals of anesthetic management involve hemodynamic control to minimize the risk of aneurysm rerupture and strategies to protect the brain against ischemic injury [(1)].

Generally, the anesthetic principles that apply to open surgical treatment of ruptured cerebral aneurysms also apply to endovascular treatment. One of the main goals of the anesthetic technique is keeping the patient motionless to optimize the quality of the images used to perform the endovascular procedure; hence, general anesthesia with endotracheal intubation is often preferred for these procedures [(1)].

Intraprocedural aneurysm rupture during endovascular treatment presents a major challenge unlike that encountered with open craniotomy. There may be a sudden and massive rise in blood pressure with or without bradycardia attributable to an elevation in intracranial pressure. Hyperventilation and osmotic diuresis may be required to control the intracranial hypertension. Aggressive treatment of surges in blood pressure may induce ischemia; therefore, antihypertensive therapy should be reserved for patients with extreme elevations in blood pressure [(1)].

Endovascular procedures differ from open procedures in that anticoagulation with heparin is frequently administered during the embolization of aneurysms. Patients who have undergone anticoagulation require rapid reversal with protamine if intraprocedural aneurysm rupture occurs. With the increasing use of intravascular stents, the administration of antiplatelet agents (aspirin, clopidogrel, and glycoprotein IIb/IIIa receptor antagonists) during these procedures has become more common. In case of intraprocedural rupture, rapid reversal of antiplatelet activity can be attempted by platelet transfusion [(1)]. The author recommends using antifibrinolytics if rupture occur during treatment. He also recommends giving antifibrinolytics immediately on arrival and until the aneurysm is obliterated.

Recommendations

1. Minimization of the degree and duration of intraoperative hypotension during aneurysm surgery is probably indicated *(Class IIa; Level of Evidence B).*
2. There are insufficient data on pharmacological strategies and induced hypertension during temporary vessel occlusion to make specific recommendations, but there are instances when their use may be considered reasonable *(Class IIb; Level of Evidence C).*
3. Induced hypothermia during aneurysm surgery is not routinely recommended but may be a reasonable option in selected cases *(Class III; Level of Evidence B).*
4. Prevention of intraoperative hyperglycemia during aneurysm surgery is probably indicated *(Class IIa; Level of Evidence B).*
5. The use of general anesthesia during endovascular treatment of ruptured cerebral aneurysms can be beneficial in selected patients *(Class IIa; Level of Evidence C).*

Management of vasospasm and DCI after aSAH

Vasospasm (narrowing) of the angiographically visible cerebral arteries after aSAH is common, occurring most frequently 7 to 10 days after aneurysm rupture and resolving spontaneously after 21 days. The cascade of events culminating in arterial narrowing is initiated when oxyhemoglobin comes in contact with the abluminal side of the vessel [(1)].

DCI is a major cause of death and disability in patients with aSAH. The management of aSAH-induced vasospasm is complex. DCI prevention include the use of oral nimodipine and maintenance of euvolemia, as well as treatment with triple-H therapy (hemodynamic augmentation therapy) and / or endovascular therapy with vasodilators and balloon angioplasty [(1)].

The use of intrathecal thrombolytic infusions could reduce the incidence and ischemic consequences of aSAH-induced vasospasm. Statin agents are commonly used also but data are conflicting [1].

Serial neurological examinations are important to detect DCI but of limited value in poor clinical grade. Along with TCD, perfusion imaging can detect hypoperfusion and may be more accurate for identification of DCI than anatomic imaging of arterial narrowing or changes in blood flow velocity by transcranial Doppler (TCD) [1].

When DCI is diagnosed, the initial treatment is the induction of hemodynamic augmentation to improve cerebral perfusion. Traditionally, hemodynamic augmentation has consisted of hemodilution (a common occurrence in this population), hypervolemia, and hypertensive (triple-H) therapy. Accumulating literature has shifted the focus from this triple-H therapy to the maintenance of euvolemia and induced hypertension [1].

Endovascular intervention is often used in patients who do not improve with hemodynamic augmentation and those with sudden focal neurological deficits and focal lesions on angiography referable to their symptoms. Interventions generally consist of balloon angioplasty for accessible lesions and vasodilator infusion for more distal vessels. Many different vasodilators (mainly calcium channel blockers) are in use. Papaverine is used less frequently because it can produce neurotoxicity. The primary limitation of vasodilator therapy is the short duration of benefit. As with hemodynamic augmentation, there are no randomized trials of these interventions, but large case series have demonstrated angiographic and clinical improvement [1].

Recommendations

1. Oral nimodipine should be administered to all patients with aSAH *(Class I; Level of Evidence A).*
2. Maintenance of euvolemia and normal circulating blood volume is recommended to prevent DCI *(Class I; Level of Evidence B).*
3. Prophylactic hypervolemia or balloon angioplasty before the development of angiographic spasm is not recommended *(Class III; Level of Evidence B).*
4. Transcranial Doppler (TCD) is reasonable to monitor for the development of arterial vasospasm *(Class IIa; Level of Evidence B).*
5. Perfusion imaging with CT or magnetic resonance can be useful to identify regions of potential brain ischemia *(Class IIa; Level of Evidence B).*
6. Induction of hypertension is recommended for patients with DCI unless blood pressure is elevated at baseline or cardiac status precludes it *(Class I; Level of Evidence B).*
7. Cerebral angioplasty and/or selective intra-arterial vasodilator therapy is reasonable in patients with symptomatic cerebral vasospasm, particularly those who are not rapidly responding to hypertensive therapy *(Class IIa; Level of Evidence B).*

▪ Management of hydrocephalus associated with aSAH

Acute hydrocephalus occurs in 15% to 87% of aSAH. Chronic shunt-dependent hydrocephalus occurs in 8.9% to 48%. Acute hydrocephalus associated with aSAH is usually managed by external ventricular drainage (EVD) or lumbar drainage. EVD is used more commonly than lumbar drain and is generally associated with neurological improvement. The risk of non-treated ruptured aneurysm rebleeding with EVD cannot be ruled out [(1)].

With lumbar drain, there is theoretical risk of tissue shift after placement of a lumbar drain in patients with severe intracranial hypertension particularly in patients with associated intraparenchymal hematomas. When obstructive hydrocephalus is suspected, an EVD should be preferred [1].

Chronic hydrocephalus associated with aSAH is usually treated with ventricular shunt placement [1].

Recommendations

1. aSAH-associated acute symptomatic hydrocephalus should be managed by cerebrospinal fluid diversion (EVD or lumbar drainage, depending on the clinical scenario) *(Class I; Level of Evidence B).*
2. aSAH-associated chronic symptomatic hydrocephalus should be treated with permanent cerebrospinal fluid diversion *(Class I; Level of Evidence C).*
3. Weaning EVD over >24 hours does not appear to be effective in reducing the need for ventricular shunting *(Class III; Level of Evidence B).*
4. Routine fenestration of the lamina terminalis is not useful for reducing the rate of shunt-dependent hydrocephalus and therefore should not be routinely performed. *(Class III; Level of Evidence B).*

Management of seizures associated with aSAH

Almost 26% of aSAH patients experience seizure-like episodes, but it remains unclear whether these episodes are verifiably epileptic in origin. More recent retrospective reviews suggest a lower seizure incidence of 6% to 18%. Delayed seizures occurred in 3% to 7% of patients. Risk factors for early seizures are aneurysm in the middle cerebral artery, thickness of aSAH clot, intracerebral hematoma, rebleeding, infarction, poor neurological grade, and history of hypertension. There is significantly lower incidence of seizures in patients treated with endovascular coiling [1].

Nonconvulsive status epilepticus is a very strong predictor of a poor outcome. Short-term prophylactic antiepileptic therapy is commonly used in patients with aSAH, based on the argument that seizures in acutely ill patients with aSAH could lead to additional injury or rebleeding from an unsecured aneurysm [1].

Recommendations

1. The use of prophylactic anticonvulsants may be considered in the immediate posthemorrhagic period *(Class IIb; Level of Evidence B).*
2. The routine long-term use of anticonvulsants is not recommended (*Class III; Level of Evidence B*) but may be considered for patients with known risk factors for delayed seizure disorder, such as prior seizure, intracerebral hematoma, intractable hypertension, infarction, or aneurysm at the middle cerebral artery *(Class IIb; Level of Evidence B).*

▪ Management of medical complications associated with aSAH

Both hypernatremia and hyponatremia are frequently observed in the acute phase after aSAH. Hyponatremia occurs in 10% to 30%. Hyponatremia has been chronologically associated with the onset of sonographic and clinical vasospasm [1].

Cerebral Salt Wasting (CSW)

CSW syndrome results from excessive secretion of natriuretic peptides and causes hyponatremia from excessive natriuresis, which may also provoke volume contraction. Occurrence of cerebral salt wasting is more common in patients with poor clinical grade, ruptured anterior communicating artery aneurysms, and hydrocephalus, and it may be an independent risk factor for poor outcome. Aggressive volume resuscitation can ameliorate the effect of cerebral salt wasting on the risk of cerebral ischemia after aSAH. 3% saline solution is effective in correcting hyponatremia. Fludrocortisones can correct hyponatremia and fluid balance and reduce need for fluids [(1)].

Fever

Fever is the most common medical complication in aSAH. The presence of fever of noninfectious (central) origin has been associated with severity of injury, amount of hemorrhage, and development of vasospasm, and it may represent a marker of a systemic inflammatory state triggered by blood and its byproducts. Improved functional outcome with effective control of fever has been reported [(1)].

Hyperglycemia

Effective glucose control after aSAH can significantly reduce the risk of poor outcome [(1)].

Anemia

Anemia is common after aSAH and may compromise brain oxygen delivery. Higher hemoglobin values are associated with improved outcomes after aSAH. The optimal hemoglobin goal after aSAH is not yet known [(1)]. The author recommends keeping Hgb > 9 especially with vasospasm.

HIT and DVT

Two additional medical complications are heparin-induced thrombocytopenia (HIT) and deep venous thrombosis (DVT). Patients with HIT type II appear to have higher rates of thrombotic complications and symptomatic vasospasm/DCI, more deaths, and significantly less favorable outcomes. It is clearly important to recognize this complication to avoid further heparin exposure and to use instead a nonheparin alternative under the guidance of a hematologist [1].

When treating medical complications, clinicians can follow the medical treatment (including anticoagulation reversal) guidelines discussed in ICH management in chapter 13.

Recommendations

1. Administration of large volumes of hypotonic fluids and intravascular volume contraction is not recommended after aSAH *(Class III; Level of Evidence B).*
2. Monitoring volume status in certain patients with recent aSAH by some combination of central venous pressure, pulmonary wedge pressure, and fluid balance is reasonable, as is treatment of volume contraction with crystalloid or colloid fluids *(Class IIa; Level of Evidence B).*
3. Aggressive control of fever to a target of normothermia by use of standard or advanced temperature modulating systems is reasonable in the acute phase of aSAH *(Class IIa; Level of Evidence B).*
4. Careful glucose management with strict avoidance of hypoglycemia may be considered as part of the general critical care management of patients with aSAH *(Class IIb; Level of Evidence B).*
5. The use of packed red blood cell transfusion to treat anemia might be reasonable in patients with aSAH who are at risk of cerebral ischemia. The optimal hemoglobin goal is still to be determined *(Class IIb; Level of Evidence B).*
6. The use of fludrocortisone acetate and hypertonic saline solution is reasonable for preventing and correcting hyponatremia *(Class IIa; Level of Evidence B).*

7. Heparin-induced thrombocytopenia and deep venous thrombosis are relatively frequent complications after aSAH. Early identification and targeted treatment are recommended, but further research is needed to identify the ideal screening paradigms *(Class I; Level of Evidence B).*

Reference

1. *Guidelines for the Management of Aneurysmal Subarachnoid Hemorrhage A Guideline for Healthcare Professionals From the American Heart Association/American Stroke Association.* E. Sander ConnollyJr, Alejandro A. Rabinstein , J. Ricardo Carhuapoma. s.l. : Stroke, 2012, Vol. 43.

15

Management of Unruptured Intracranial Aneurysms (UIAs)

▪ Epidemiology

Unruptured intracranial aneurysms (UIAs) are found in ~3.2% of population (mean age 50 years). They are being discovered incidentally with an increasing frequency because of the widespread use of high-resolution magnetic resonance imaging (MRI) scanning. The large majority of UIAs will never rupture. Prevalence over-all is higher in people aged ≥30 years [1].

▪ Risk factors

IA risk can be divided into factors associated with 3 phases: 1) risk for aneurysm development; 2) risk for growth or morphological change; and 3) risk for rupture. IAs are acquired lesions and are the cause of most cases (80%–85%) of nontraumatic SAH; however, the proportion of IAs that rupture is unknown [1]. Please refer to table 10.2 for strength and level of evidence while reading guidelines and recommendations.

Nonmodifiable Risk Factors

There is increasing frequency by age, with a peak in the fifth and sixth decade of age. When aneurysms are found in children they are usually associated with other conditions or genetic risk. There is an increased frequency of IAs in women compared with men, with aneurysms occurring more frequently in women across the age spectrum [1].

At-Risk Disorders

There is an increased risk of aneurysm formation in disorders such as polycystic kidney disease, type IV Ehlers-Danlos syndrome, Marfan syndrome, coarctation of the aorta, bicuspid aortic valve, pseudoxanthoma elasticum, hereditary hemorrhagic telangiectasia, neurofibromatosis type 1, α_1-antitrypsin deficiency, fibromuscular dysplasia, pheochromocytoma, Klinefelter syndrome, tuberous sclerosis, Noonan syndrome, α-glucosidase deficiency, microcephalic osteodysplastic primordial dwarfism, and intracranial arteriovenous malformations [1].

Family History and Genetics

7% to 20% of aneurysms are familial. There is also higher chance (4%) of harboring aneurysms in first-degree relatives (especially siblings) of patients with SAH. There are many factors that increase chance of familial aneurysms such as older age, female sex, cigarette smoking, history of hypertension, higher lipid levels, higher fasting glucose, family history of polycystic kidney disease, and family history of SAH or aneurysm in ≥2 relatives [1].

The inheritance patterns of IAs are unclear, but autosomal dominance transmission is suspected to be the most common mode of inheritance. A variety of genes or chromosomal regions have been identified in both familial and sporadic cases of IAs [(1)].

Modifiable Risk Factors

Current and former (to lesser extent) smokers are at risk of IA. Hypertension is considered a risk factor for development and rupture of aneurysms. Excessive alcohol use is considered risk factor for aneurysm development. The role of oral contraceptives has been controversial in aSAH [(1)].

Multiplicity

Two or more aneurysms are found in 15% to 30% of patients. Risk factors for multiple aneurysms include female sex, cigarette smoking, hypertension, a family history of cerebrovascular disease, and postmenopausal hormone replacement therapy [(1)].

Risk Factors for Aneurysmal Change

Growth

Aneurysm growth can result from increased blood pressure, hemodynamic stress based on location and shape of the aneurysm, and inflammation. A variety of factors for growth that have been identified include female sex, cigarette smoking, younger age, excessive alcohol consumption, aneurysm location, multiplicity of aneurysms and history of SAH, stroke and TIA. Other risk factors that contribute to growth are initial aneurysm size and arterial branch–related aneurysms [(1)].

Predictors

In addition to traditional factors such as aneurysm size and location, there are many other risk factors for aneurysm growth and rupture. Other risk factors include younger age, cigarette smoking, hypertension, aneurysmal growth, morphology, female sex, prior SAH, and family history of SAH. Inflammation may play an important role in the pathogenesis and growth of IAs. The role of anti-inflammatory medications in prevention of growth and rupture is not well established. Aspirin use could lead to fewer SAH events [1]. Also refer to PHASES score in chapter 2, table 2.6.

Recommendations

1. Given that smoking appears to increase the risk of UIA formation, patients with UIA should be counseled regarding the importance of smoking cessation *(Class I; Level of Evidence B)*.
2. Given that hypertension may play a role in growth and rupture of IAs, patients with UIA should monitor blood pressure and undergo treatment for hypertension *(Class I; Level of Evidence B)*.
3. Aneurysmal growth may increase the risk of rupture, and intermittent imaging studies to follow those UIAs managed conservatively should be considered *(Class I; Level of Evidence B)*.

▪ Clinical presentation

UIAs are most commonly (~30%) identified after hemorrhage from another aneurysm, or incidentally during evaluation of neurological symptoms such as headache (23.7%), ischemic cerebrovascular disease or transient ischemic attack (10.6% and 10.5%), cranial nerve palsy (8.0%), seizures (2.9%), mass effect (2.7%), subdural or intracerebral hemorrhage (1.2%), brain tumor (0.8%), central nervous system degenerative disorders

(0.4%), and undefined "spells" (7.1%). There is ~4-fold increased risk of rupture with symptomatic unruptured aneurysms [1].

When UIAs are discovered due to resultant cranial nerve palsy, there is likely chance of imminent rupture (especially with 3rd nerve palsy) and improvement in cranial nerve function after aneurysm treatment [1].

Recommendations

1. Patients with an aSAH should undergo careful assessment for a coexistent UIA *(Class I; Level of Evidence B)*.
2. Early treatment is generally indicated for patients presenting with cranial nerve palsy caused by a UIA *(Class I; Level of Evidence C)*.
3. The effectiveness of the routine treatment of UIAs for the prevention of ischemic cerebrovascular disease is uncertain *(Class IIb; Level of Evidence C)*.

▪ Diagnosis/Imaging

MRA, CTA, and DSA are used in diagnosing UIA. Each has advantages and disadvantages, and each is used variably by individual practitioners at various stages in the evaluation of cerebral aneurysms [1].

After the diagnosis of an aneurysm, the specific anatomic (and perhaps in the future, dynamic) details of the aneurysm(s) both initially and in follow-up are necessary to adequately categorize the lesion to select appropriate management and assess the outcomes of that management [1].

Digital Subtraction Angiography (DSA)

DSA is the "gold standard" of aneurysm diagnosis; however, with the advent of 3-dimensional (3D) rotational angiography, even more detailed imaging can be performed than with 2-dimensional planar imaging. In general, the risks from DSA are low, with most contemporary data indicating permanent neurological complications in patients with cerebral aneurysms, SAH, and arteriovenous malformation occurring at a rate of 0.07%. The potential radiation risks are small. Selective DSA follow-up for treated aneurysms also carries a low risk [(1)].

Computed Tomography Angiography (CTA)

CTA is considered the initial diagnostic test of choice for aneurysm detection and screening. CTA has sensitivity of 93.3% and specificity of 87.8% compared with DSA. In addition, CT is very useful in identifying mural calcification and thrombus, which can have a significant impact on treatment decisions. However, the reconstruction methods may not accurately depict the true neck/dome/adjacent small vessel anatomy, which can be important determinates of the type of treatment rendered [(1)].

CTA may be limited by artifact from bone and metal (coils, stents, and clips), thereby reducing its usefulness as an alternative to DSA as a follow-up technique for noninvasive imaging in treated aneurysms. The associated exposure to radiation is another issue in its use in long-term follow-up [(1)].

Magnetic Resonance Angiogram (MRA)

The MRA technique that is typically used for aneurysms assessment is time-of-flight (TOF) or contrast methods. MRA has sensitivity ranging from 74% to 98% especially with aneurysms >3 mm. These data suggest that as a primary method of screening for UIAs, magnetic resonance can be very useful for aneurysms larger than 3 mm [1].

For follow-up after interventional treatment, although susceptibility artifacts occur at the skull base and surrounding metallic implants such as stents, coils, and clips, MRA remains an effective alternative for noninvasive follow-up of both treated and untreated aneurysms [1].

MRA is preferred over CTA or DSA if there is concern in individual patients about ionizing radiation or contrast [1].

Analysis and Reporting

With adequate clipping, often no follow-up imaging is performed, or it may be limited to immediate peri-operative angiography. For endovascularly treated aneurysms, because a residual or recurrent aneurysm is more common, imaging is often performed at 6 months to 1 year after treatment. Timing of the later follow-ups is variable and depends on the occlusion status of the initial and early follow-up, as well as the condition of the patient. However, with residual aneurysms after coiling, long-term follow-up is indicated because there are late hemorrhages and aneurysm recurrences. For example, annual rates of hemorrhage in large and giant aneurysms (the most difficult group to treat with coiling) are up to 1.9%. There is evidence that certain characteristics, such as wider neck diameters, larger aneurysms, and partial treatment, have a greater association with recurrence [1].

Recommendations

1. DSA can be useful compared with noninvasive imaging for identification and evaluation of cerebral aneurysms if surgical or endovascular treatment is being considered *(Class IIa; Level of Evidence B)*.

2. DSA is reasonable as the most sensitive imaging for follow-up of treated aneurysms *(Class IIa; Level of Evidence C).*
3. CTA and MRA are useful for detection and follow- up of UIA *(Class I; Level of Evidence B).*
4. It is reasonable to perform MRA as an alternative for follow-up for treated aneurysms, with DSA used as necessary when deciding on therapy *(Class IIa; Level of Evidence C).*
5. Coiled aneurysms, especially those with wider neck or dome diameters or those that have residual filling, should have follow-up evaluation *(Class I; Level of Evidence B).* The timing and duration of follow-up is uncertain, and additional investigation is necessary.
6. The importance of surveillance imaging after endovascular treatment of UIAs lacking high-risk features for recurrence remains unclear, but surveillance imaging is probably indicated *(Class IIa; Level of Evidence C).*

▪ Screening

Screening for unruptured aneurysms is appropriate in the following cases: 1) families with >1 affected person with an IA, especially smokers and hypertensive with 2 affected siblings or ≥3 affected family members ; 2) patients with a family history of IA and evidence of autosomal dominant polycystic kidney disease, type IV Ehlers-Danlos (vascular subtype), 3) coarctation of the aorta or bicuspid aortic valve, 4) first-degree relatives of those with SAH [1].

Recommendations

1. Patients with ≥2 family members with IA or SAH should be offered aneurysmal screening by CTA or MRA. Risk factors that predict a particularly high risk of aneurysm occurrence in such families include history of hypertension, smoking, and female sex *(Class I; Level of Evidence B).*
2. Patients with a history of autosomal dominant polycystic kidney disease, particularly those with a family history of IA, should be offered screening by CTA or MRA *(Class I; Level of Evidence B),* and it is

reasonable to offer CTA or MRA to patients with coarctation of the aorta and patients with microcephalic osteodysplastic primordial dwarfism *(Class IIa; Level of Evidence B)*.

Natural history of UIAs

Among patients with no history of SAH, the rupture risk was 0.05% per year for aneurysms <10 mm in diameter and ~ 1% per year for larger aneurysms; aneurysm size and location in the posterior or posterior communicating artery were predictors of rupture risk in this group [(1)]. The PHASES score (Table 2.6) and Table 15.1 summarize the most important risk factors.

Table 15.1. Risk of aneurysm rupture based on size and location

Five-Year Cumulative Rupture Rates (%) According to Size and Location of Unruptured Aneurysm					
	Group 1 <7 mm	**Group 2 <7 mm**	**7-12 mm**	**13-24 mm**	**>24 mm**
Cavernous carotid artery	0	0	0	3.0	6.4
AC/MC/IC	0	1.5	2.6	14.5	40
Post-P Com	2.5	3.4	14.5	18.4	50
AC indicates anterior communicating or anterior cerebral artery; IC, internal carotid artery (not cavernous carotid artery); MC, middle cerebral artery; and Post-P comm, vertebrobasilar, posterior cerebral arterial system, or the posterior communicating artery.					

Routine screening by noninvasive vascular imaging techniques to detect aneurysm growth is probably indicated, and treatment of aneurysms with documented growth may be reasonable.

Recommendations

1. Prior history of aSAH may be considered to be an independent risk factor for future hemorrhage secondary to a different small unruptured aneurysm *(Class IIb; Level of Evidence B).*
2. Patients with aneurysms with documented enlargement during follow-up should be offered treatment in the absence of prohibitive comorbidities *(Class I; Level of Evidence B).*
3. Treatment of UIAs in patients with a family history of IA is reasonable even in aneurysms at smaller sizes than spontaneously occurring IAs *(Class IIa; Level of Evidence B).*

▪ Surgical clipping

The first obliterative clipping of an aneurysm was performed by Walter Dandy in 1938. Since then many surgical techniques have developed.

Surgical Techniques [2]

Ipsilateral Simple Clipping

Two principles apply in surgical clipping: isolating the lesion from active circulation and maintaining the integrity and patency of the parenting vessel. The key to successful clipping lies in good neck exposure, and in cases where visual exposure and clip insertion is limited by the operating field, endoscope-assisted clipping can be used [2].

Contralateral Access for MCA Aneurysm

This technique is used when MCA aneurysm is within a short distance from the midline, especially if aneurysm is pointing toward the midline. It is preferable when dealing with bilateral MCA aneurysms needing treatment to save patient from a second craniotomy [2].

Temporary Artery Occlusion (TAO)

TAO allows the aneurysm to shrink, offering the operator better vision and space to operate while preventing rupture. TAO is applied only for 10 to 20 minutes to prevent ischemia. TAO is still one of the most widely used techniques in clipping surgeries [2].

Microscope-Integrated Near-Infrared Indocyanine Green Video Angiography (ICGVA)

ICGVA is used to assess real-time intraoperative patency of parenting vessel and perforator [2].

Wrapping and Clipping

Wrapping and clipping is a technique applied to ruptured aneurysms where the lesion is wrapped with autogenous tissue or absorbable material to reconstruct the integrity of the vessel wall before clipping. However, this method is not suitable for complete neck avulsion due to the deficit aneurysmal neck or residual root; in such cases an in-situ bypass is required [2].

Bypass Techniques

Extracranial-to-intracranial (EC-IC) Bypass

Low-flow EC-IC bypass involves the superficial temporal artery (STA) to an intracranial artery (STA-IC). This technique is used for giant aneurysms to bypass flow around the aneurysm and relieve mass effect [(2)].

High-flow EC-IC bypass involves the common carotid artery (CCA) or external carotid artery (ECA) to an intracranial artery (CCA-IC or ECA-IC). High-flow bypass is not preferable due to potential hyperperfusion damage [(2)].

Intracranial-to-Intracranial (IC-IC) Bypass

There are 4 common sites in the cerebral circulation that are anatomically suitable for IC-IC bypass: 1) the ACAs, A2 and A3 segments, as they course over the genu and rostrum of the corpus callosum; 2) the MCA branches, through the sylvian fissure; 3) the posterior cerebral artery (PCA) and superior cerebellar artery, the section around midbrain through ambient cistem; and 4) the posterior ICAs (PICAs), around the posterior medulla and the tonsils in cisterna magna. It is recommended for bister aneurysm where parent artery sacrifice is the only solution to prevent bleeding [(2)].

Bipolar Coagulating for Microaneurysms

Microaneurysms do not require aggressive surgery. In cases where surgery is inevitable, such as recurrent SAH, clipping is not suitable for their miniature nature; instead, direct bipolar coagulating is highly effective. It is important to differentiate small BBAs from microaneurysms. While they resemble each other on imaging and other characteristics, direct bipolar coagulating of BBAs can lead to massive bleeding.

Efficacy and Durability

Although surgical clipping is believed to provide definitive and long-term treatment of aneurysms; however, there is limited data available regarding the long-term risk of intracranial hemorrhage after UIA clipping. There is a need for continued follow-up in patients with known residua after clipping. Due to risk of de novo aneurysms it warrants consideration for repeat imaging within a 5- to 10-year time frame, and even up to 20 years in younger patients.

Risk Factors: Lesion Specific

The size and location of aneurysms have been most consistently associated with surgical risk. Non-giant (<25 mm) anterior circulation aneurysms carried the lowest mortality estimate of 0.8% (1.9% morbidity) compared with non-giant posterior circulation aneurysms at 3% (12.9% morbidity), giant anterior circulation aneurysms at 7.4% (26.9% morbidity), and giant posterior circulation aneurysms at 9.6% (37.9% morbidity).

Other aneurysm features, such as atheroma/calcification, thrombus, non-saccular morphology, and multiplicity, pose additional challenges and have been reported to adversely affect surgical outcome.

Risk Factors: Patient Specific

Older age and deep location of aneurysms are the important risk factor influencing outcomes after surgical clipping. Also, clipping ruptured aneurysms and higher SAH grade carry higher risk than non-ruptured aneurysms and lower grade SAH. History of prior ischemic cerebrovascular disease is associated with a significantly higher risk for adverse events after clipping. There is also strong volume-outcome relationship related to outcomes after aneurysm surgery for both UIA and RIA in the United States [(1)].

Recommendations

1. Several factors, including patient age and aneurysm location and size, should be taken into account when considering surgical clipping as the mode of treatment for a UIA *(Class I; Level of Evidence B).*
2. Imaging after surgical intervention, to document aneurysm obliteration, is recommended given the differential risk of growth and hemorrhage for completely versus incompletely obliterated aneurysms *(Class I; Level of Evidence B).*
3. Long-term follow-up imaging may be considered after surgical clipping given the combined risk of aneurysm recurrence and de novo aneurysm formation. Long-term follow-up may be particularly important for those aneurysms that are incompletely obliterated during initial treatment *(Class IIb; Level of Evidence B).*
4. Surgical treatment of UIA is recommended to be performed at higher-volume centers (eg, performing >20 cases annually) *(Class I; Level of Evidence B).*
5. The use of specialized intraoperative tools and techniques for avoiding vessel compromise or residual aneurysms may be considered to reduce the adverse outcomes seen with operative management of UIAs *(Class IIb; Level of Evidence C).*

Endovascular Treatment

Guglielmi invented the endovascular approach using electrolytically detachable coils in 1991.

Endovascular Techniques

Simple Coiling

Simple coiling refers to transluminal navigation of a microcatheter into the aneurysmal dome with the help of micro guidewires and the delivery and packing of detachable coils within the aneurysmal sac. This promotes clot formation within the aneurysmal sac, hence isolating it from active circulation.

Simple coiling is suitable for all IAs with desirable dome-to-neck ratios (>2.0), excluding blister aneurysms as their fragile wall poses high risks of perforation [2].

Double Catheter Technique

Two microcatheters are positioned in the proximal and distal aspects of the aneurysmal dome. The first coil is deployed proximal to create a supporting frame, and then the rest of the coils are deposited via the distal microcatheter. The framing coil is not detached until satisfactory packing is obtained. This technique is used if dome-to-neck ratio (≤2.0, >1.5). This technique is safe and effective for elongated IAs, especially for those at MCA bifurcations [2].

Balloon-Assisted Coiling (BAC)

BAC is used in treating IAs with a wide neck and unfavorable dome-to-neck ratio (≤1.5, >1.0) [2]. BAC involves placement of the deflated balloon catheter across the neck of the aneurysm and a microcatheter within the sac of the aneurysm. The balloon is inflated when coil prolapse, and this is repeated with every coil placement and before detachment.

Stent-Assisted Coiling (SAC) [2]

SAC involves deploying a stent to block the neck before coil packing. The SAC is used with wide-necked, gigantic, fusiform, and some other complex aneurysms especially with dome-to-neck ratio (≤1.0). There are 4 major SAC techniques:

Simple (mesh) SAC: A stent is deployed as the first step and then a microcatheter is navigated into the aneurysmal lumen via the mesh of the stent.

Stent jail SAC: The microcatheter is positioned before the stent bridging over the aneurysmal neck.

Stent jack SAC: The stent is deployed after the deployment of the first coil in the aneurysmal sac.

Y-stenting SAC: It is used for bifurcation aneurysm, where 2 stents are deployed blocking the aneurysmal neck.

Flow-Diverting Stent (FDS)

FDSs are a new generation of stents designed to treat aneurysm by isolating the aneurysmal lumen from the circulation via recanalization. The FDSs are suitable for both wide-necked and fusiform aneurysms. They are either braided mesh stents, such as the Silk Flow Diverter (Balt Extrusion, Montmorency, France), the Pipeline Embolization Device (ev3, Irvine, California), or covered stents such as the Willis Covered Stent (MicroPort Medical Company, Shanghai, China) [2].

Overall, endovascular aneurysm repair is the preferred treatment in many medical centers. Due to better outcomes for endovascular coil occlusion of ruptured aneurysms than for surgical clipping in selected cases. Technical failure rates range between 0% and 10%. Complications occur in 5% to 10% of cases (1).

Despite that there is risk of aneurysm recanalization after endovascular occlusion; however, the recurrent hemorrhage rate is low. The likelihood of aneurysm recanalization appears greater in previously ruptured aneurysms than in unruptured aneurysms (1).

For unruptured aneurysms, recanalization of bifurcation aneurysms after endovascular coil occlusion remains a problem, especially at the middle cerebral bifurcation and at the carotid and basilar artery termini, although recanalization can also occur with clipped aneurysms at lower rates [(1)].

Recommendations

1. Endoluminal flow diversion represents a new treatment strategy that may be considered in carefully selected cases *(Class IIb; Level of Evidence B)*. Other emerging technologies to treat unruptured cerebral aneurysms, such as liquid embolic agents, represent new treatment strategies that may be considered in carefully selected cases *(Class IIb; Level of Evidence C)*. The long-term effects of these newer approaches remain largely unknown. Strict adherence to the US Food and Drug Administration's indications for use is probably indicated until additional trial data demonstrate an incremental improvement in safety and efficacy over existing technologies *(Class IIa; Level of Evidence C)*.
2. Use of coated coils is not beneficial compared with bare-metal coils *(Class III; Level of Evidence A)*.
3. Endovascular treatment of UIAs is recommended to be performed at high-volume centers *(Class I; Level of Evidence B)*.
4. The procedural risk of radiation exposure should be explicitly reviewed in the consent process for endovascular procedures *(Class I; Level of Evidence C)*.

Aneurysm follow-up (untreated)

Recommendations

1. For patients with UIAs that are managed noninvasively without either surgical or endovascular intervention, radiographic follow-up with MRA or CTA at regular intervals is indicated. The optimal

interval and duration of recommended follow-up are uncertain *(Class I; Level of Evidence B)*.

2. For patients with UIAs that are managed noninvasively without either surgical or endovascular intervention, a first follow-up study at 6 to 12 months after initial discovery, followed by subsequent yearly or every other year follow-up, may be reasonable *(Class IIb; Level of Evidence C)*.
3. For patients with UIAs that are managed noninvasively and in whom there are no contraindications to MRI, it may be reasonable to consider TOF MRA rather than CTA for repeated long-term follow-up *(Class IIb; Level of Evidence C)*.

Overall recommendations

1. Several factors should be considered in selection of the optimal management of a UIA, including the size, location, and other morphological characteristics of the aneurysm; documented growth on serial imaging; the age of the patient; a history of prior aSAH; family history of cerebral aneurysm; the presence of multiple aneurysms; or the presence of concurrent pathology such as an arteriovenous malformation or other cerebrovascular or inherited pathology that may predispose to a higher risk of hemorrhage *(Class I; Level of Evidence C)*.
2. Patients with unruptured cerebral aneurysms who are considered for treatment should be fully informed about the risks and benefits of both endovascular and micro- surgical treatment as alternatives to secure the UIAs and prevent bleeding *(Class I; Level of Evidence B)*.
3. The results of UIA treatment are inferior at low-volume centers, and hence treatment is recommended to be performed at higher-volume centers *(Class I; Level of Evidence B)*.
4. Data from prospective and retrospective studies from multiple national and international investigations indicate that microsurgical clip ligation may confer more durable protection against aneurysm regrowth, but coil embolization may be superior to surgical clipping with respect to procedural morbidity and mortality, length of stay, and hospital costs, so it may be reasonable to choose endovascular

therapy over surgical clipping in the treatment of select UIAs, particularly in cases for which surgical morbidity is high, such as at the basilar apex and in the elderly *(Class IIb; Level of Evidence B).*

5. The treatment risk of patients with UIAs is related to advancing age, medical comorbidities, and aneurysm location and size, so in older patients (>65 years of age) and those with associated medical comorbidities with small asymptomatic UIAs and low hemorrhage risk by location, size, morphology, family history, and other relevant factors, observation is a reasonable alternative *(Class IIa; Level of Evidence B).*

References

1. *Guidelines for the Management of Patients With Unruptured Intracranial Aneurysms.* B. Gregory Thompson, Robert D. BrownJr , Sepideh Amin-Hanjani. s.l. : Stroke, 2015, Vol. 46.
2. *Current Treatment Strategies for Intracranial Aneurysms: An Overview.* Junjie Zhao, MD, MSc, Hao Lin, MD, Richard Summers, MSc. 1, s.l. : Angiology, 2018, Vol. 69.

16

Stroke Prevention Guidelines (1)

The main purpose of this book is to mainly address acute stroke management. However, due to necessity to implement some preventive measures in the acute phase, the author devoted this chapter to stroke prevention guidelines that standardize the management of stroke risk factors.

Annual recurrent stroke rate is 3%–4%. This rate is decreasing due to the use of antiplatelet therapy and effective strategies for treatment of hypertension, atrial fibrillation (AF), arterial obstruction, and hyperlipidemia.

Although prevention of ischemic stroke is the primary outcome of interest, many of the grades for the recommendations were chosen to reflect the existing evidence on the reduction of all vascular outcomes after stroke or TIA, including subsequent stroke, myocardial infarction (MI), and vascular death. Please refer to table 10.2 for strength and level of evidence while reading guidelines and recommendations.

▪ Hypertension (HTN)

1. Initiation of blood pressure (BP) therapy is indicated for previously untreated patients with ischemic stroke or TIA who,

after the first several days, have an established BP ≥140 mm Hg systolic or ≥90 mm Hg diastolic *(Class I; Level of Evidence B)*. Initiation of therapy for patients with BP <140 mm Hg systolic and <90 mm Hg diastolic is of uncertain benefit *(Class IIb; Level of Evidence C)*.

2. Resumption of BP therapy is indicated for previously treated patients with known HTN for both prevention of recurrent stroke and prevention of other vascular events in those who have had an ischemic stroke or TIA and are beyond the first several days *(Class I; Level of Evidence A)*.

3. Goals for target BP level or reduction from pretreatment baseline are uncertain and should be individualized, but it is reasonable to achieve a systolic pressure <140 mm Hg and a diastolic pressure <90 mm Hg *(Class IIa; Level of Evidence B)*. For patients with a recent lacunar stroke, it might be reasonable to target a systolic blood pressure (SBP) of <130 mm Hg *(Class IIb; Level of Evidence B)*.

4. Several lifestyle modifications have been associated with BP reductions and are a reasonable part of a comprehensive antihypertensive therapy *(Class IIa; Level of Evidence C)*. These modifications include salt restriction; weight loss; the consumption of a diet rich in fruits, vegetables, and low-fat dairy products; regular aerobic physical activity; and limited alcohol consumption.

5. The optimal drug regimen to achieve the recommended level of reductions is uncertain because direct comparisons between regimens are limited. The available data indicate that diuretics or the combination of diuretics and an angiotensin-converting enzyme inhibitor is useful *(Class I; Level of Evidence A)*.

6. The choice of specific drugs and targets should be individualized on the basis of pharmacological properties, mechanism of action, and consideration of specific patient

characteristics for which specific agents are probably indicated (eg, extracranial cerebrovascular occlusive disease, renal impairment, cardiac disease, and diabetes mellitus [DM]) *(Class IIa; Level of Evidence B).*

▪ Dyslipidemia (DLP)

1. Statin therapy with intensive lipid-lowering effects is recommended to reduce risk of stroke and cardiovascular events among patients with ischemic stroke or TIA presumed to be of atherosclerotic origin and low-density lipoprotein cholesterol (LDL-C) level ≥100 mg/dL with or without evidence for other clinical atherosclerotic cardiovascular disease (ASCVD) *(Class I; Level of Evidence B).*
2. Statin therapy with intensive lipid-lowering effects is recommended to reduce risk of stroke and cardiovascular events among patients with ischemic stroke or TIA presumed to be of atherosclerotic origin, an LDL-C level <100 mg/dL, and no evidence for other clinical ASCVD *(Class I; Level of Evidence C).*
3. Patients with ischemic stroke or TIA and other comorbid ASCVD should be otherwise managed according to the 2013 ACC/AHA cholesterol guidelines, which include lifestyle modification, dietary recommendations, and medication recommendations *(Class I; Level of Evidence A).*

▪ Diabetes mellitus (DM)

1. After a TIA or ischemic stroke, all patients should probably be screened for DM with testing of fasting plasma glucose, HbA_{1c}, or an oral glucose tolerance test. Choice of test and timing should be guided by clinical judgment and recognition that acute illness may temporarily perturb measures of plasma glucose. In general, HbA_{1c} may be more accurate than other

screening tests in the immediate post event period *(Class IIa; Level of Evidence C).*

2. Use of existing guidelines from the American Diabetes Association for glycemic control and cardiovascular risk factor management is recommended for patients with an ischemic stroke or TIA who also have DM or pre-DM *(Class I; Level of Evidence B).*

Obesity

1. All patients with TIA or stroke should be screened for obesity with measurement of body mass index *(Class I; Level of Evidence C).*

2. Despite the demonstrated beneficial effects of weight loss on cardiovascular risk factors, the usefulness of weight loss among patients with a recent TIA or ischemic stroke and obesity is uncertain *(Class IIb; Level of Evidence C).*

Metabolic syndrome

1. At this time, the usefulness of screening patients for the metabolic syndrome after stroke is unknown *(Class IIb; Level of Evidence C).*

2. For patients who are screened and classified as having the metabolic syndrome, management should focus on counseling for lifestyle modification (diet, exercise, and weight loss) for vascular risk reduction *(Class I; Level of Evidence C).*

3. Preventive care for patient with the metabolic syndrome should include appropriate treatment for individual components of the syndrome, which are also stroke risk factors, particularly dyslipidemia and HTN *(Class I; Level of Evidence A).*

▪ Physical inactivity

1. For patients with ischemic stroke or TIA who are capable of engaging in physical activity, at least 3 to 4 sessions per week of moderate- to vigorous-intensity aerobic physical exercise are reasonable to reduce stroke risk factors. Sessions should last an average of 40 minutes. Moderate- intensity exercise is typically defined as sufficient to break a sweat or noticeably raise heart rate (eg, walking briskly, using an exercise bicycle). Vigorous-intensity exercise includes activities such as jogging *(Class IIa; Level of Evidence C).*
2. For patients who are able and willing to initiate increased physical activity, referral to a comprehensive, behaviorally oriented program is reasonable *(Class IIa; Level of Evidence C).*
3. For individuals with disability after ischemic stroke, supervision by a healthcare professional such as a physical therapist or cardiac rehabilitation professional, at least on initiation of an exercise regimen, may be considered *(Class IIb; Level of Evidence C).*

▪ Nutrition

1. It is reasonable to conduct a nutritional assessment for patients with a history of ischemic stroke or TIA, looking for signs of overnutrition or undernutrition *(Class IIa; Level of Evidence C).*
2. Patients with a history of ischemic stroke or TIA and signs of undernutrition should be referred for individualized nutritional counseling *(Class I; Level of Evidence B).*
3. Routine supplementation with a single vitamin or combination of vitamins is not recommended *(Class III; Level of Evidence A).*
4. It is reasonable to recommend that patients with a history of stroke or TIA reduce their sodium intake to less than ≈2.4 g/d.

Further reduction to <1.5 g/d is also reasonable and is associated with even greater BP reduction *(Class IIa; Level of Evidence C)*.

5. It is reasonable to counsel patients with a history of stroke or TIA to follow a Mediterranean-type diet instead of a low-fat diet. The Mediterranean-type diet emphasizes vegetables, fruits, and whole grains and includes low-fat dairy products, poultry, fish, legumes, olive oil, and nuts. It limits intake of sweets and red meats *(Class IIa; Level of Evidence C)*.

▪ Sleep apnea

1. A sleep study might be considered for patients with an ischemic stroke or TIA on the basis of the very high prevalence of sleep apnea in this population and the strength of the evidence that the treatment of sleep apnea improves outcomes in the general population *(Class IIb; Level of Evidence B)*.
2. Treatment with continuous positive airway pressure might be considered for patients with ischemic stroke or TIA and sleep apnea given the emerging evidence in support of improved outcomes *(Class IIb; Level of Evidence B)*.

▪ Cigarette smoking

1. Healthcare providers should strongly advise every patient with stroke or TIA who has smoked in the past year to quit *(Class I; Level of Evidence C)*.
2. It is reasonable to advise patients after TIA or ischemic stroke to avoid environmental (passive) tobacco smoke *(Class IIa; Level of Evidence B)*.

3. Counseling, nicotine products, and oral smoking cessation medications are effective in helping smokers to quit *(Class I; Level of Evidence A).*

▪ Alcohol consumption

1. Patients with ischemic stroke, TIA, or hemorrhagic stroke who are heavy drinkers should eliminate or reduce their consumption of alcohol *(Class I; Level of Evidence C).*

2. Light to moderate amounts of alcohol consumption (up to 2 drinks per day for men and up to 1 drink per day for nonpregnant women) may be reasonable, although nondrinkers should not be counseled to start drinking *(Class IIb; Level of Evidence B).*

▪ Extracranial carotid disease

1. For patients with a TIA or ischemic stroke within the past 6 months and ipsilateral severe (70%–99%) carotid artery stenosis as documented by noninvasive imaging, carotid endarterectomy (CEA) is recommended if the perioperative morbidity and mortality risk is estimated to be <6% *(Class I; Level of Evidence A).*

2. For patients with recent TIA or ischemic stroke and ipsilateral moderate (50%–69%) carotid stenosis as documented by catheter-based imaging or noninvasive imaging with corroboration (eg, magnetic resonance angiogram or computed tomography angiogram), CEA is recommended depending on patient-specific factors, such as age, sex, and comorbidities, if the perioperative morbidity and mortality risk is estimated to be <6% *(Class I; Level of Evidence B).*

3. When the degree of stenosis is <50%, CEA and carotid angioplasty and stenting (CAS) are not recommended *(Class III; Level of Evidence A)*

4. When revascularization is indicated for patients with TIA or minor, nondisabling stroke, it is reasonable to perform the procedure within 2 weeks of the index event rather than delay surgery if there are no contraindications to early revascularization *(Class IIa; Level of Evidence B)*.

5. CAS is indicated as an alternative to CEA for symptomatic patients at average or low risk of complications associated with endovascular intervention when the diameter of the lumen of the internal carotid artery is reduced by >70% by noninvasive imaging or >50% by catheter-based imaging or noninvasive imaging with corroboration and the anticipated rate of periprocedural stroke or death is <6% *(Class IIa; Level of Evidence B)*.

6. It is reasonable to consider patient age in choosing between CAS and CEA. For older patients (ie, older than ≈70 years), CEA may be associated with improved outcome compared with CAS, particularly when arterial anatomy is unfavorable for endovascular intervention. For younger patients, CAS is equivalent to CEA in terms of risk for periprocedural complications (ie, stroke, MI, or death) and long-term risk for ipsilateral stroke *(Class IIa; Level of Evidence B)*.

7. Among patients with symptomatic severe stenosis (>70%) in whom anatomic or medical conditions are present that greatly increase the risk for surgery or when other specific circumstances exist such as radiation-induced stenosis or

restenosis after CEA, CAS is reasonable *(Class IIa; Level of Evidence B).*

8. CAS and CEA in the above settings should be performed by operators with established periprocedural stroke and mortality rates of <6% for symptomatic patients, similar to that observed in trials comparing CEA to medical therapy and more recent observational studies *(Class I; Level of Evidence B).* Routine, long-term follow-up imaging of the extracranial carotid circulation with carotid duplex ultrasonography is not recommended *(Class III; Level of Evidence B).*

9. For patients with a recent (within 6 months) TIA or ischemic stroke ipsilateral to a stenosis or occlusion of the middle cerebral or carotid artery, extracranial/intra-cranial (EC/IC) bypass surgery is not recommended *(Class III; Level of Evidence A).*

1. For patients with recurrent or progressive ischemic symptoms ipsilateral to a stenosis or occlusion of a distal (surgically inaccessible) carotid artery, or occlusion of a midcervical carotid artery after institution of optimal medical therapy, the usefulness of EC/IC bypass is considered investigational *(Class IIb; Level of Evidence C).*

2. Optimal medical therapy, which should include antiplatelet therapy, statin therapy, and risk factor modification, is recommended for all patients with carotid artery stenosis and a TIA or stroke, as outlined elsewhere in this guideline *(Class I; Level of Evidence A).*

Extracranial vertebrobasilar disease

1. Routine preventive therapy with emphasis on antithrombotic therapy, lipid lowering, BP control, and lifestyle optimization is

recommended for all patients with recently symptomatic extracranial vertebral artery stenosis *(Class I; Level of Evidence C)*.

2. Endovascular stenting of patients with extracranial vertebral stenosis may be considered when patients are having symptoms despite optimal medical treatment *(Class IIb; Level of Evidence C)*.
3. Open surgical procedures, including vertebral endarterectomy and vertebral artery transposition, may be considered when patients are having symptoms despite optimal medical treatment *(Class IIb; Level of Evidence C)*.

Intracranial atherosclerosis

1. For patients with a stroke or TIA caused by 50% to 99% stenosis of a major intracranial artery, aspirin 325 mg/d is recommended in preference to warfarin *(Class I; Level of Evidence B)*.
2. For patients with recent stroke or TIA (within 30 days) attributable to severe stenosis (70%–99%) of a major intracranial artery, the addition of clopidogrel 75 mg/d to aspirin for 90 days might be reasonable *(Class IIb; Level of Evidence B)*.
3. For patients with stroke or TIA attributable to 50% to 99% stenosis of a major intracranial artery, the data are insufficient to make a recommendation regarding the usefulness of clopidogrel alone, the combination of aspirin and dipyridamole, or cilostazol alone *(Class IIb; Level of Evidence C)*.
4. For patients with a stroke or TIA attributable to 50% to 99% stenosis of a major intracranial artery, maintenance of SBP below 140 mm Hg and high-intensity statin therapy are recommended *(Class I; Level of Evidence B)*.
5. For patients with a stroke or TIA attributable to moderate stenosis (50%–69%) of a major intracranial artery, angioplasty or stenting is not recommended given the low rate of stroke with medical management and the inherent periprocedural risk of endovascular treatment *(Class III; Level of Evidence B)*.

6. For patients with stroke or TIA attributable to severe stenosis (70%–99%) of a major intracranial artery, stenting with the Wingspan stent system is not recommended as an initial treatment, even for patients who were taking an antithrombotic agent at the time of the stroke or TIA *(Class III; Level of Evidence B)*.

7. For patients with stroke or TIA attributable to severe stenosis (70%–99%) of a major intracranial artery, the usefulness of angioplasty alone or placement of stents other than the Wingspan stent is unknown and is considered investigational *(Class IIb; Level of Evidence C)*.

8. For patients with severe stenosis (70%–99%) of a major intracranial artery and recurrent TIA or stroke after institution of aspirin and clopidogrel therapy, achievement of SBP <140 mmHg, and high-intensity statin therapy, the usefulness of angioplasty alone or placement of a Wingspan stent or other stent is unknown and is considered investigational *(Class IIb; Level of Evidence C)*.

9. For patients with severe stenosis (70%–99%) of a major intracranial artery and actively progressing symptoms after institution of aspirin and clopidogrel therapy, the usefulness of angioplasty alone or placement of a Wingspan stent or other stents is unknown and is considered investigational *(Class IIb; Level of Evidence C)*.

10. For patients with stroke or TIA attributable to 50% to 99% stenosis of a major intracranial artery, EC/IC bypass surgery is not recommended *(Class III; Level of Evidence B)*.

▪ Atrial fibrillation

1. For patients who have experienced an acute ischemic stroke or TIA with no other apparent cause, prolonged rhythm monitoring (≈30 days) for atrial fibrillation (AF) is reasonable

within 6 months of the index event *(Class IIa; Level of Evidence C).*

2. Vitamin K antagonist (VKA) therapy *(Class I; Level of Evidence A)*, apixaban *(Class I; Level of Evidence A)*, and dabigatran *(Class I; Level of Evidence B)* are all indicated for the prevention of recurrent stroke in patients with nonvalvular AF, whether paroxysmal or permanent. The selection of an antithrombotic agent should be individualized on the basis of risk factors, cost, tolerability, patient preference, potential for drug interactions, and other clinical characteristics, including renal function and time in international normalized ratio (INR) therapeutic range if the patient has been taking VKA therapy.
3. Rivaroxaban is reasonable for the prevention of recurrent stroke in patients with nonvalvular AF *(Class IIa; Level of Evidence B).*
4. For patients with ischemic stroke or TIA with paroxysmal (intermittent), persistent, or permanent AF in whom VKA therapy is begun, a target INR of 2.5 is recommended (range, 2.0–3.0) *(Class I; Level of Evidence A).*
5. The combination of oral anticoagulation (ie, warfarin or one of the newer agents) with antiplatelet therapy is not recommended for all patients after ischemic stroke or TIA but is reasonable in patients with clinically apparent coronary artery disease, particularly an acute coronary syndrome or stent placement *(Class IIb; Level of Evidence C).*
6. For patients with ischemic stroke or TIA and AF who are unable to take oral anticoagulants, aspirin alone is recommended *(Class I; Level of Evidence A)*. The addition of clopidogrel to aspirin therapy, compared with aspirin therapy alone, might be reasonable *(Class IIb; Level of Evidence B).*
7. For most patients with a stroke or TIA in the setting of AF, it is reasonable to initiate oral anticoagulation within 14 days after the onset of neurological symptoms *(Class IIa; Level of Evidence B).*

8. In the presence of high risk for hemorrhagic conversion (ie, large infarct, hemorrhagic transformation on initial imaging, uncontrolled HTN, or hemorrhage tendency), it is reasonable to delay initiation of oral anticoagulation beyond 14 days *(Class IIa; Level of Evidence B)*.

9. For patients with AF and a history of stroke or TIA who require temporary interruption of oral anticoagulation, bridging therapy with low-molecular-weight heparin (LMWH) (or equivalent anticoagulant agent if intolerant to heparin) is reasonable, depending on perceived risk for thromboembolism and bleeding *(Class IIa; Level of Evidence C)*.

1. The usefulness of closure of the left atrial appendage with the WATCHMAN device in patients with ischemic stroke or TIA and AF is uncertain *(Class IIb; Level of Evidence B)*.

Acute MI and left ventricular thrombus

1. Treatment with VKA therapy (target INR, 2.5; range, 2.0–3.0) for 3 months is recommended in most patients with ischemic stroke or TIA in the setting of acute MI complicated by left ventricular (LV) mural thrombus formation identified by echocardiography or another imaging modality *(Class I; Level of Evidence C)*. Additional antiplatelet therapy for cardiac protection may be guided by recommendations such as those from the American College of Chest Physicians.

2. Treatment with VKA therapy (target INR, 2.5; range, 2.0–3.0) for 3 months may be considered in patients with ischemic stroke or TIA in the setting of acute anterior ST-segment MI without demonstrable LV mural thrombus formation but with anterior apical akinesis or dyskinesis identified by echocardiography or other imaging modality *(Class IIb; Level of Evidence C)*.

3. In patients with ischemic stroke or TIA in the setting of acute MI complicated by LV mural thrombus formation or anterior or apical wall-motion abnormalities with an LV ejection fraction <40% who are intolerant to VKA therapy because of nonhemorrhagic adverse events, treatment with an LMWH, dabigatran, rivaroxaban, or apixaban for 3 months may be considered as an alternative to VKA therapy for prevention of recurrent stroke or TIA *(Class IIb; Level of Evidence C).*

▪ Cardiomyopathy

1. In patients with ischemic stroke or TIA in sinus rhythm who have left atrial or LV thrombus demonstrated by echocardiography or another imaging modality, anticoagulant therapy with a VKA is recommended for ≥3 months *(Class I; Level of Evidence C).*
2. In patients with ischemic stroke or TIA in the setting of a mechanical LV assist device, treatment with VKA therapy (target INR, 2.5; range, 2.0–3.0) is reasonable in the absence of major contraindications (eg, active gastrointestinal bleeding) *(Class IIa; Level of Evidence C).*
3. In patients with ischemic stroke or TIA in sinus rhythm with either dilated cardiomyopathy (LV ejection fraction ≤35%) or restrictive cardiomyopathy without evidence of left atrial or LV thrombus, the effectiveness of anti- coagulation compared with antiplatelet therapy is uncertain, and the choice should be individualized *(Class IIb; Level of Evidence B).*
4. In patients with ischemic stroke or TIA in sinus rhythm with dilated cardiomyopathy (LV ejection fraction ≤35%), restrictive cardiomyopathy, or a mechanical LV assist device who are intolerant to VKA therapy because of nonhemorrhagic adverse events, the effectiveness of treatment with dabigatran,

rivaroxaban, or apixaban is uncertain compared with VKA therapy for prevention of recurrent stroke *(Class IIb; Level of Evidence C)*.

Mitral stenosis, regurgitation, prolapse and annular calcification, and aortic valve disease

1. For patients with ischemic stroke or TIA who have rheumatic mitral valve disease and AF, long-term VKA therapy with an INR target of 2.5 (range, 2.0–3.0) is recommended *(Class I; Level of Evidence A)*.
2. For patients with ischemic stroke or TIA who have rheumatic mitral valve disease without AF or another likely cause for their symptoms (eg, carotid stenosis), long-term VKA therapy with an INR target of 2.5 (range, 2.0–3.0) may be considered instead of antiplatelet therapy *(Class IIb; Level of Evidence C)*.
3. For patients with rheumatic mitral valve disease who are prescribed VKA therapy after an ischemic stroke or TIA, antiplatelet therapy should not be routinely added *(Class III; Level of Evidence C)*.
4. For patients with rheumatic mitral valve disease who have an ischemic stroke or TIA while being treated with adequate VKA therapy, the addition of aspirin might be considered *(Class IIb; Level of Evidence C)*.
5. For patients with ischemic stroke or TIA and native aortic or nonrheumatic mitral valve disease who do not have AF or another indication for anticoagulation, antiplatelet therapy is recommended *(Class I; Level of Evidence C)*.
6. For patients with ischemic stroke or TIA and mitral annular calcification who do not have AF or another indication for anticoagulation, antiplatelet therapy is recommended as it

would be without the mitral annular calcification *(Class I; Level of Evidence C).*

7. For patients with mitral valve prolapse who have ischemic stroke or TIAs and who do not have AF or another indication for anticoagulation, antiplatelet therapy is recommended as it would be without mitral valve prolapse *(Class I; Level of Evidence C).*

Prosthetic heart valve

1. For patients with a mechanical aortic valve and a history of ischemic stroke or TIA before its insertion, VKA therapy is recommended with an INR target of 2.5 (range, 2.0–3.0) *(Class I; Level of Evidence B).*
2. For patients with a mechanical mitral valve and a history of ischemic stroke or TIA before its insertion, VKA therapy is recommended with an INR target of 3.0 (range, 2.5–3.5) *(Class I; Level of Evidence C).*
3. For patients with a mechanical mitral or aortic valve who have a history of ischemic stroke or TIA before its insertion and who are at low risk for bleeding, the addition of aspirin 75 to 100 mg/d to VKA therapy is recommended *(Class I; Level of Evidence B).*
4. For patients with a mechanical heart valve who have an ischemic stroke or systemic embolism despite adequate antithrombotic therapy, it is reasonable to intensify therapy by increasing the dose of aspirin to 325 mg/d or increasing the target INR, depending on bleeding risk *(Class IIa; Level of Evidence C).*
5. For patients with a bioprosthetic aortic or mitral valve, a history of ischemic stroke or TIA before its insertion, and no other indication for anticoagulation therapy beyond 3 to 6 months from the valve placement, long-term therapy with aspirin 75 to

100 mg/d is recommended in preference to long-term anticoagulation *(Class I; Level of Evidence C).*

6. For patients with a bioprosthetic aortic or mitral valve who have a TIA, ischemic stroke, or systemic embolism despite adequate antiplatelet therapy, the addition of VKA therapy with an INR target of 2.5 (range, 2.0–3.0) may be considered *(Class IIb; Level of Evidence C).*

Antiplatelet agent

1. For patients with noncardioembolic ischemic stroke or TIA, the use of antiplatelet agents rather than oral anti- coagulation is recommended to reduce the risk of recur- rent stroke and other cardiovascular events *(Class I; Level of Evidence A).*
2. Aspirin (50–325 mg/d) monotherapy (*Class I; Level of Evidence A*) or the combination of aspirin 25 mg and extended-release dipyridamole 200 mg twice daily *(Class I; Level of Evidence B)* is indicated as initial therapy after TIA or ischemic stroke for prevention of future stroke.
3. Clopidogrel (75 mg) monotherapy is a reasonable option for secondary prevention of stroke in place of aspirin or combination aspirin/dipyridamole *(Class IIa; Level of Evidence B).* This recommendation also applies to patients who are allergic to aspirin.
4. The selection of an antiplatelet agent should be individualized on the basis of patient risk factor profiles, cost, tolerance, relative known efficacy of the agents, and other clinical characteristics *(Class I; Level of Evidence C).*
5. The combination of aspirin and clopidogrel might be considered for initiation within 24 hours of a minor ischemic stroke or TIA and for continuation for 21 days *(Class IIb; Level of Evidence B).*
6. The combination of aspirin and clopidogrel, when initiated days to years after a minor stroke or TIA and continued for 2 to 3

years, increases the risk of hemorrhage relative to either agent alone and is not recommended for routine long-term secondary prevention after ischemic stroke or TIA *(Class III; Level of Evidence A)*.

7. For patients who have an ischemic stroke or TIA while taking aspirin, there is no evidence that increasing the dose of aspirin provides additional benefit. Although alternative antiplatelet agents are often considered, no single agent or combination has been adequately studied in patients who have had an event while receiving aspirin *(Class IIb; Level of Evidence C)*.
8. For patients with a history of ischemic stroke or TIA, AF, and coronary artery disease, the usefulness of adding antiplatelet therapy to VKA therapy is uncertain for purposes of reducing the risk of ischemic cardiovascular and cerebrovascular events *(Class IIb; Level of Evidence C)*. Unstable angina and coronary artery stenting represent special circumstances in which management may warrant dual antiplatelet therapy / VKA therapy.

Oral anticoagulant

1. For patients with noncardioembolic ischemic stroke or TIA, the use of antiplatelet agents rather than oral anticoagulation is recommended to reduce the risk of recurrent stroke and other cardiovascular events *(Class I; Level of Evidence A)*.

Aortic arch atheroma

1. For patients with an ischemic stroke or TIA and evidence of aortic arch atheroma, antiplatelet therapy is recommended *(Class I; Level of Evidence A)*.

2. For patients with an ischemic stroke or TIA and evidence of aortic arch atheroma, statin therapy is recommended *(Class I; Level of Evidence B)*.
3. For patients with ischemic stroke or TIA and evidence of aortic arch atheroma, the effectiveness of anticoagulation with warfarin, compared with antiplatelet therapy, is unknown *(Class IIb; Level of Evidence C)*.
4. Surgical endarterectomy of aortic arch plaque for the purposes of secondary stroke prevention is not recommended *(Class III; Level of Evidence C)*.

Arterial dissection

1. For patients with ischemic stroke or TIA and extracranial carotid or vertebral arterial dissection, antithrombotic treatment with either antiplatelet or anticoagulant therapy for at least 3 to 6 months is reasonable *(Class IIa; Level of Evidence B)*.
2. The relative efficacy of antiplatelet therapy compared with anticoagulation is unknown for patients with ischemic stroke or TIA and extracranial carotid or vertebral arterial dissection *(Class IIb; Level of Evidence B)*.
3. For patients with stroke or TIA and extracranial carotid or vertebral arterial dissection who have definite recurrent cerebral ischemic events despite medical therapy, endovascular therapy (stenting) may be considered *(Class IIb; Level of Evidence C)*.
4. Patients with stroke or TIA and extracranial carotid or vertebral arterial dissection who have definite recurrent cerebral ischemic events despite medical therapy and also fail or are not candidates for endovascular therapy may be considered for surgical treatment *(Class IIb; Level of Evidence C)*.

▪ Patent foramen ovale (PFO)

1. There are insufficient data to establish whether anticoagulation is equivalent or superior to aspirin for secondary stroke prevention in patients with patent foramen ovale (PFO) *(Class IIb; Level of Evidence B)*.
2. For patients with an ischemic stroke or TIA and a PFO who are not undergoing anticoagulation therapy, antiplatelet therapy is recommended *(Class I; Level of Evidence B)*.
3. For patients with an ischemic stroke or TIA and both a PFO and a venous source of embolism, anticoagulation is indicated, depending on stroke characteristics *(Class I; Level of Evidence A)*. When anticoagulation is contraindicated, an inferior vena cava filter is reasonable *(Class IIa; Level of Evidence C)*.
4. For patients with a cryptogenic ischemic stroke or TIA and a PFO without evidence for deep vein thrombosis (DVT) available data do not support a benefit for PFO closure *(Class III; Level of Evidence A)*.
5. In the setting of PFO and DVT, PFO closure by a transcatheter device might be considered, depending on the risk of recurrent DVT *(Class IIb; Level of Evidence C)*.

▪ Hyperhomocysteinemia

1. Routine screening for hyperhomocysteinemia among patients with a recent ischemic stroke or TIA is not indicated *(Class III; Level of Evidence C)*.
2. In adults with a recent ischemic stroke or TIA who are known to have mild to moderate hyperhomocysteinemia, supplementation with folate, vitamin B_6, and vitamin B_{12} safely

reduces levels of homocysteine but has not been shown to prevent stroke *(Class III; Level of Evidence B).*

Hypercoagulable states

1. The usefulness of screening for thrombophilic states in patients with ischemic stroke or TIA is unknown *(Class IIb; Level of Evidence C).*
2. Anticoagulation might be considered in patients who are found to have abnormal findings on coagulation testing after an initial ischemic stroke or TIA, depending on the abnormality and the clinical circumstances *(Class IIb; Level of Evidence C).*
3. Antiplatelet therapy is recommended for patients who are found to have abnormal findings on coagulation testing after an initial ischemic stroke or TIA if anticoagulation therapy is not administered *(Class I; Level of Evidence A).*
4. Long-term anticoagulation might be reasonable for patients with spontaneous cerebral venous sinus thrombosis or a recurrent ischemic stroke of undefined origin and an inherited thrombophilia *(Class IIb; Level of Evidence C).*

Antiphospholipid antibodies

1. Routine testing for antiphospholipid antibodies is not recommended for patients with ischemic stroke or TIA who have no other manifestations of the antiphospholipid antibody syndrome (APS) and who have an alternative explanation for their ischemic event, such as atherosclerosis, carotid stenosis, or AF *(Class III; Level of Evidence C).*
2. For patients with ischemic stroke or TIA who have an antiphospholipid antibody but do not fulfill the criteria for APS,

antiplatelet therapy is recommended *(Class I; Level of Evidence B).*

3. For patients with ischemic stroke or TIA who meet the criteria for the APS, anticoagulant therapy might be considered depending on the perception of risk for recurrent thrombotic events and bleeding *(Class IIb; Level of Evidence C).*
4. For patients with ischemic stroke or TIA who meet the criteria for the APS but in whom anticoagulation is not begun, antiplatelet therapy is indicated *(Class I; Level of Evidence A).*

▪ Sickle cell disease

1. For patients with sickle cell disease and prior ischemic stroke or TIA, chronic blood transfusions to reduce hemoglobin S to <30% of total hemoglobin are recommended *(Class I; Level of Evidence B).*
2. For patients with sickle cell disease and prior ischemic stroke or TIA for whom transfusion therapy is not available or practical, treatment with hydroxyurea may be considered *(Class IIb; Level of Evidence B).*
3. For adults with sickle cell disease and ischemic stroke or TIA, general treatment recommendations cited else- where in this guideline are reasonable with regard to the control of risk factors and the use of antiplatelet agents *(Class IIa; Level of Evidence B).*

▪ Cerebral venous sinus thrombosis

1. Anticoagulation is reasonable for patients with acute cerebral venous sinus thrombosis, even in selected patients with intracranial hemorrhage *(Class IIa; Level of Evidence B).*

2. In cerebral venous sinus thrombosis patients without a recognized thrombophilia, it is reasonable to administer anticoagulation for ≥3 months, followed by antiplatelet therapy *(Class IIa; Level of Evidence C)*. Recommendations for patients with a recognized thrombophilia are discussed elsewhere in this document.

▪ Pregnancy

1. In the presence of a high-risk condition that would require anticoagulation outside of pregnancy, the following options are reasonable:

   a. LMWH twice daily throughout pregnancy, with dose adjusted to achieve the LMWH manufacturer's recommended peak anti-Xa activity 4 hours after injection, or
   b. Adjusted-dose unfractionated heparin (UFH) throughout pregnancy, administered subcutaneously every 12 hours in doses adjusted to keep the midinterval activated partial thromboplastin time at least twice control or to maintain an anti-Xa heparin level of 0.35 to 0.70 U/mL, or
   c. UFH or LMWH (as above) until the 13th week, followed by substitution of a VKA until close to delivery, when UFH or LMWH is resumed. (Class IIa; Level of Evidence C).

2. For pregnant women receiving adjusted-dose LMWH therapy for a high-risk condition that would require anticoagulation outside of pregnancy, and when delivery is planned, it is reasonable to discontinue LMWH ≥24 hours before induction of labor or cesarean section *(Class IIa; Level of Evidence C).*

3. In the presence of a low-risk situation in which antiplatelet therapy would be the treatment recommendation outside of pregnancy, UFH or LMWH, or no treatment may be considered during the first trimester of pregnancy depending on the clinical situation *(Class IIb; Level of Evidence C).*

4. In the presence of a low-risk situation in which antiplatelet therapy would be the treatment recommendation outside of pregnancy, low-dose aspirin (50–150 mg/d) is reasonable after the first trimester of pregnancy *(Class IIa; Level of Evidence B)*.

Breastfeeding women

1. In the presence of a high-risk condition that would require anticoagulation outside of pregnancy, it is reasonable to use warfarin, UFH, or LMWH *(Class IIa; Level of Evidence C)*.
2. In the presence of a low-risk situation in which antiplatelet therapy would be the treatment recommendation outside of pregnancy, low-dose aspirin use may be considered *(Class IIb; Level of Evidence C)*.

Anticoagulation after ICH

1. The decision to restart antithrombotic therapy after intracranial hemorrhage (ICH) related to antithrombotic therapy depends on the risk of subsequent arterial or venous thromboembolism, the risk of recurrent ICH, and the overall status of the patient and must therefore be individualized to each patient. For patients with a comparatively lower risk of cerebral infarction (eg, AF without prior ischemic stroke) and a higher risk of recurrent ICH (eg, elderly patients with lobar ICH or presumed amyloid angiopathy) or with very poor overall neurological function, an antiplatelet agent may be considered for prevention of ischemic stroke *(Class IIb; Level of Evidence B)*.
2. For patients who require resumption or initiation of anticoagulation after an acute ICH, subarachnoid hemorrhage,

or subdural hematoma, the optimal timing is uncertain. For most patients, however, it might be reasonable to wait ≥1 week *(Class IIb; Level of Evidence B)*.

3. For patients with hemorrhagic cerebral infarction, continuation of anticoagulation may be considered, depending on the specific clinical scenario and underlying indication for anticoagulant therapy *(Class IIb; Level of Evidence C)*.

▪ Special approaches in high-risk populations

1. Monitoring achievement of nationally accepted, evidence-based guidelines on a population-based level is recommended as a basis for improving health-promotion behaviors and reducing stroke healthcare disparities among high-risk groups *(Class I; Level of Evidence C)*.
2. Voluntary hospital-based programs for quality monitoring and improvement are recommended to improve adherence to nationally accepted, evidence-based guidelines for secondary stroke prevention *(Class I; Level of Evidence C)*.

References

1. *Guidelines for the Prevention of Stroke in Patients With Stroke and Transient Ischemic Attack.* Walter N. Kernan, MD, Chair, Bruce Ovbiagele, MD, MSc, MAS, Vice Chair and Henry R. Black, MD. s.l. : Stroke, 2014, Vol. 45.

Abbreviations

AC	anti-coagulation
ACA	anterior cerebral artery
ACHA	anterior choroidal artery
ACOMA	anterior communicating artery
ACS	acute coronary syndrome
AF	atrial fibrillation
AICA	anterior inferior cerebellar artery
AIS	acute ischemic stroke
AMS	altered mental status
ASA	American Stroke Association
ASRH	acute stroke ready hospital
AVM	arteriovenous malformation
BA	basilar artery
BTO	balloon occlusion test
CAA	cerebral amyloid angiopathy
CAD	cervical atherosclerotic disease
CAS	carotid angioplasty and stenting
CBF	cerebral blood flow
CC	collateral circulation
CCA	common carotid artery
CEA	carotid endarterectomy
CIN	contrast-induced nephropathy
CNS	central nervous system
CPP	cerebral perfusion pressure
CPSS	Cincinnati Prehospital Stroke Scale
CSC	comprehensive stroke center
CSF	cerebrospinal fluid
CSW	cerebral salt wasting
CT	computed tomography
CTA	CT angiogram
CTP	CT perfusion
CVP	central venous pressure
CVR	cerebrovascular resistance
CVT	cerebral venous thrombosis
DAP	dual anti-platelet
DBP	diastolic blood pressure
DC	decompressive craniectomy
DCI	delayed cerebral ischemia
DM	diabetes mellitus
DOAC	direct oral anti-coagulant
DSA	digital subtraction angiography
DVT	deep venous thrombosis
DWI	diffusion-weighted imaging
ECA	external carotid artery
ED	emergency department
EDH	epidural hemorrhage
EEG	electroencephalography
EMS	emergency medical services
EVD	external ventricular drainage
EVT	endovascular treatment
FAST	**F**acial droop, **A**rm weakness, and **S**peech difficulty, and if these deficits are found, it's **T**ime to call 9-1-1
FDA	Food and Drug Administration
GCS	Glasgow Coma Scale

HE	hematoma evacuation
HIT	heparin-induced thrombocytopenia
HT	hemorrhagic transformation
HTN	hypertension
IA	intraarterial
ICAD	intra-cranial atherosclerotic disease
ICA	internal carotid artery
ICH	intracerebral hemorrhage
ICP	intracranial pressure
INR	international normalized ratio
ISU	inpatient stroke unit
IVH	intraventricular hemorrhage
IV tPA	intravenous tissue plasminogen activator
LAPSS	Los Angeles Prehospital Stroke Screen
LKW	last known well
LMWH	low-molecular-weight heparin
LOC	level of consciousness
LV	left ventricle
MAP	mean arterial pressure
MCA	middle cerebral artery
MENDC	Miami Emergency Neurologic Deficit Checklist
MI	myocardial infarction
MISE	minimally invasive surgical evacuation
MRA	magnetic resonance angiogram
MRI	magnetic resonance image
mRS	modified Rankin Scale
NAS	neuro-angiography suite
NCCT	non-contrast CT
NICU	neuro intensive care unit
NIH	National Institutes of Health
NIHSS	National Institute of Health Stroke Scale
NI	neurointerventional
OA	ophthalmic artery
PCA	posterior cerebral artery
PC-AKI	Post Contrast Acute Kidney Injury
PCOMA	posterior communication artery
PSC	primary stroke center
PE	pulmonary embolism
PFO	patent foramen ovale
PNS	peripheral nervous system
POCT	point of care testing
SAH	subarachnoid hemorrhage
SBP	systolic blood pressure
SCA	superior cerebellar artery
SDH	subdural hemorrhage
SNIS	Society of Neurointerventional Surgery
SVS	small vessel (lacunar) stroke
TCD	transcranial Doppler
TCSC	thrombectomy capable stroke center
TIA	transient ischemic attack
UFH	unfractionated heparin
UIA	unruptured intracranial aneurysm
VA	vertebral artery
VC	ventricular catheter
VKA	vitamin K antagonist
VTE	venous thromboembolism

72738868R00174

Made in the USA
Columbia, SC
01 September 2019